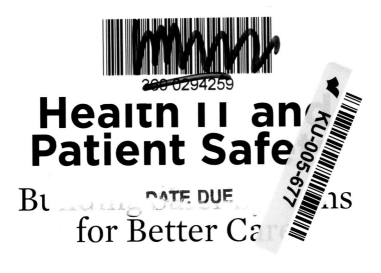

Health IT and Patient Safety

Building Safer Systems for Better Care

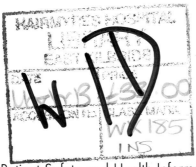

Committee on Patient Safety and Health Information Technology

Board on Health Care Services

INSTITUTE OF MEDICINE
OF THE NATIONAL ACADEMIES

THE NATIONAL ACADEMIES PRESS
Washington, D.C.
www.nap.edu

THE NATIONAL ACADEMIES PRESS   500 Fifth Street, NW   Washington, DC 20001

NOTICE: The project that is the subject of this report was approved by the Governing Board of the National Research Council, whose members are drawn from the councils of the National Academy of Sciences, the National Academy of Engineering, and the Institute of Medicine. The members of the committee responsible for the report were chosen for their special competences and with regard for appropriate balance.

This study was supported by Contract No. HHSP23337018T between the National Academy of Sciences and the United States Department of Health and Human Services. Any opinions, findings, conclusions, or recommendations expressed in this publication are those of the author(s) and do not necessarily reflect the view of the organizations or agencies that provided support for this project.

Library of Congress Cataloging-in-Publication Data

Institute of Medicine (U.S.). Committee on Patient Safety and Health Information Technology.
  Health IT and patient safety : building safer systems for better care / Committee on Patient Safety and Health Information Technology, Board on Health Care Services.
    p. ; cm.
  Includes bibliographical references.
  ISBN 978-0-309-22112-2 (pbk.) — ISBN 978-0-309-22113-9 (PDF)
  I. Title.
  [DNLM: 1. Health Facilities—United States. 2. Patient Safety—United States. 3. Medical Errors—prevention & control—United States. 4. Medical Informatics Applications—United States. WX 185]

  610.28'9—dc23
                         2012007111

Additional copies of this report are available from the National Academies Press, 500 Fifth Street, NW, Keck 360, Washington, DC 20001; (800) 624-6242 or (202) 334-3313; Internet, http://www.nap.edu.

For more information about the Institute of Medicine, visit the IOM home page at: **www. iom.edu.**

The serpent has been a symbol of long life, healing, and knowledge among almost all cultures and religions since the beginning of recorded history. The serpent adopted as a logotype by the Institute of Medicine is a relief carving from ancient Greece, now held by the Staatliche Museen in Berlin.

Suggested citation: IOM (Institute of Medicine). 2012. *Health IT and Patient Safety: Building Safer Systems for Better Care.* Washington, DC: The National Academies Press.

"Knowing is not enough; we must apply.
Willing is not enough; we must do."
—Goethe

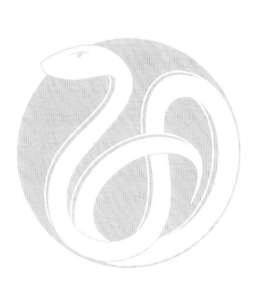

INSTITUTE OF MEDICINE
OF THE NATIONAL ACADEMIES

Advising the Nation. Improving Health.

THE NATIONAL ACADEMIES
Advisers to the Nation on Science, Engineering, and Medicine

The **National Academy of Sciences** is a private, nonprofit, self-perpetuating society of distinguished scholars engaged in scientific and engineering research, dedicated to the furtherance of science and technology and to their use for the general welfare. Upon the authority of the charter granted to it by the Congress in 1863, the Academy has a mandate that requires it to advise the federal government on scientific and technical matters. Dr. Ralph J. Cicerone is president of the National Academy of Sciences.

The **National Academy of Engineering** was established in 1964, under the charter of the National Academy of Sciences, as a parallel organization of outstanding engineers. It is autonomous in its administration and in the selection of its members, sharing with the National Academy of Sciences the responsibility for advising the federal government. The National Academy of Engineering also sponsors engineering programs aimed at meeting national needs, encourages education and research, and recognizes the superior achievements of engineers. Dr. Charles M. Vest is president of the National Academy of Engineering.

The **Institute of Medicine** was established in 1970 by the National Academy of Sciences to secure the services of eminent members of appropriate professions in the examination of policy matters pertaining to the health of the public. The Institute acts under the responsibility given to the National Academy of Sciences by its congressional charter to be an adviser to the federal government and, upon its own initiative, to identify issues of medical care, research, and education. Dr. Harvey V. Fineberg is president of the Institute of Medicine.

The **National Research Council** was organized by the National Academy of Sciences in 1916 to associate the broad community of science and technology with the Academy's purposes of furthering knowledge and advising the federal government. Functioning in accordance with general policies determined by the Academy, the Council has become the principal operating agency of both the National Academy of Sciences and the National Academy of Engineering in providing services to the government, the public, and the scientific and engineering communities. The Council is administered jointly by both Academies and the Institute of Medicine. Dr. Ralph J. Cicerone and Dr. Charles M. Vest are chair and vice chair, respectively, of the National Research Council.

www.national-academies.org

COMMITTEE ON PATIENT SAFETY AND
HEALTH INFORMATION TECHNOLOGY

PHILIP SCHNEIDER, Clinical Professor and Associate Dean, University of Arizona College of Pharmacy, Phoenix, AZ
CHRISTINE A. SINSKY, Physician, Department of Internal Medicine, Medical Associates Clinic and Health Plans, Dubuque, IA
PAUL C. TANG,[2] Vice President, Chief Innovation and Technology Officer, Palo Alto Medical Foundation and Consulting Associate Professor of Medicine, Stanford University, Stanford, CA

IOM Study Staff

SAMANTHA M. CHAO, Study Director
PAMELA CIPRIANO, Distinguished Nurse Scholar-in-Residence
HERBERT S. LIN, Chief Scientist, Computer Sciences and Telecommunications Board
JENSEN N. JOSE, Research Associate
JOI D. WASHINGTON, Research Assistant
ROGER C. HERDMAN, Director, Board on Health Care Services

---

[2] Committee member since August 2011 and special advisor to the committee prior to that.

Reviewers

This report has been reviewed in draft form by individuals chosen for their diverse perspectives and technical expertise, in accordance with procedures approved by the National Research Council's Report Review Committee. The purpose of this independent review is to provide candid and critical comments that will assist the institution in making its published report as sound as possible and to ensure that the report meets institutional standards for objectivity, evidence, and responsiveness to the study charge. The review comments and draft manuscript remain confidential to protect the integrity of the deliberative process. We wish to thank the following individuals for their review of this report:

JOHN R. CLARKE, Drexel University
JANET M. CORRIGAN, National Quality Forum
KURTIS ELWARD, University of Virginia
JOHN GLASER, Siemens Medical Solutions USA, Inc.
PETER BARTON HUTT, Covington & Burling, LLP
ROSS KOPPEL, University of Pennsylvania
GILAD KUPERMAN, New York–Presbyterian Hospital
NAJMEDIN MEHSKATI, University of Southern California
MARTYN THOMAS, Martyn Thomas Associates

Although the reviewers listed above have provided many constructive comments and suggestions, they were not asked to endorse the conclusions or recommendations, nor did they see the final draft of the report before its release. The review of this report was overseen by **ALFRED O.**

BERG, University of Washington School of Medicine, and **BRADFORD H. GRAY,** Urban Institute. Appointed by the National Research Council and Institute of Medicine, they were responsible for making certain that an independent examination of this report was carried out in accordance with institutional procedures and that all review comments were carefully considered. Responsibility for the final content of this report rests entirely with the authoring committee and the institution.

Preface

"Perfection is not attainable, but if we chase perfection we can reach excellence."

—Vince Lombardi

We are at a unique time in health care. Technology—which has the potential to improve quality and safety of care as well as reduce costs—is rapidly evolving, changing the way we deliver health care. At the same time, health care reform is reshaping the health care landscape. As Sir Cyril Chantler of the Kings Fund said, "Medicine used to be simple, ineffective, and relatively safe. Now it is complex, effective, and potentially dangerous." More and more cognitive overload requires a symbiotic relationship between human cognition and computer support. It is this very difficult transition we are facing in ensuring safety in health care.

Caught in the middle are the patients—the ultimate recipients of care. Stories of patient injuries and deaths associated with health information technologies (health IT) frequently appear in the news, juxtaposed with stories of how health professionals are being provided monetary incentives to adopt the very products that may be causing harm. These stories are frightening, but they shed light on a very important problem and a realization that, as a nation, we must do better to keep patients safe.

The committee was asked to review the evidence about the impact of health IT on patient safety and to recommend actions to be taken by both the private and public sectors. As always, Institute of Medicine (IOM) reports are to be based on the evidence. We examined the peer-reviewed literature in depth and solicited examples of harm from the public. We also specifically sought and received input from the vendor community on numerous occasions. We found that specific types of health IT can improve patient safety under the right conditions, but those conditions cannot be replicated easily and require continual effort to achieve. We tried to balance the findings in the literature with anecdotes from the field but came to the realization that the information needed for an objective analysis and assessment of the safety of health IT and its use was not available. This realization was eye-opening and drove the committee to consider ways to make information about the magnitude of the harm discoverable.

The committee offers a vision for how the discipline of safety science can be better integrated into a health IT–enabled world. Early on we concluded that safety is the product of the larger sociotechnical system and emerges from the interaction between different parts of this larger system. This finding is not new. It is apparent in many other industries and has been introduced in health care before, but it needs to be underscored.

Building on the concept of a sociotechnical system, the committee concluded that safer systems require efforts to be made by all stakeholders. A coordinated effort will be needed from the private sector. However, the public sector must also be part of a solution to protect patient safety for two reasons: (1) patient safety is a public good and (2) with the government's large investment in this area, it has a fiduciary responsibility to ensure the value of its investment.

Definitive evidence was not available in many areas, such as determining what the roles of specific private- and public-sector actors should be and how regulation would impact innovation in this area. Where evidence was not available, the committee—broad in its expertise and beliefs—relied on its expert opinion. While the entire committee believes the current state of safety of health IT must not be permitted to continue, individual approaches differed on how to best move forward and the speed for doing so. Over the course of many conversations, the committee designed recommendations that balance these approaches and strike common ground, outlining a private–public framework for improving patient safety without constraining innovation.

Unfortunately, we were unable to resolve the issues raised by one committee member. In his statement of dissent in Appendix E, he calls for health IT to be regulated as a Class III device under the Food and Drug Administration's (FDA's) medical device classification scheme. The dissent makes no mention of FDA's capacity or the very serious implications that regulation of health IT by FDA as a Class III device could have on innovation. We deliberated about these issues over the course of the entire study and tried at length to understand each other's perspectives toward reaching consensus on the issues. In Chapter 6, the committee states that we believe the impact of regulation on innovation needs to be carefully weighed. We also discuss that if regulation is necessary, FDA should consider a new, more flexible approach outside of the traditional medical device classification scheme. The committee determined that it was not within its purview to discuss details of what this approach would be. The determination of classes should be the responsibility of FDA and not of this committee.

As chair, I would like to personally thank the members of the committee for their time, effort, and willingness to engage in these discussions. I also want to thank the IOM staff for their work in guiding the committee through this process.

The committee hopes actions that follow the release of this report will in a few years give us a better sense of both risks and remedies for application of health IT in the field. As the nation continues to move forward in adopting health IT, we must act with urgency to protect the safety of patients.

Gail L. Warden, *Chair*
Committee on Patient Safety and
Health Information Technology
August 2011

Acknowledgments

The committee and staff would like to thank those who presented statements and presentations at the public workshops held on December 14, 2010, in Washington, DC, and on February 24, 2011, in Irvine, California:

Cameron Anderson, Family Healthcare Network
Karen Bell, Certification Commission for Health Information Technology
Kenneth Chrisman, Wells Fargo Bank, NA
Darren Dworkin, Cedars-Sinai
Floyd Eisenberg, National Quality Forum
Scott Finley, Westat
Ellen Harper, Cerner
Rainu Kaushal, Cornell University
Nancy Leveson, Massachusetts Institute of Technology
William Munier, Agency for Healthcare Research and Quality
Mary Beth Navarra-Sirio, McKesson
Don Norman, Nielsen Norman Group
Judy Ozbolt, Westat
Steven Palmer, Family Healthcare Network
Peter Pronovost, Johns Hopkins University
Sumit Rana, Epic
Madhu Reddy, Pennsylvania State University
Ben Shneiderman, University of Maryland
Lawrence Shulman, Dana-Farber Cancer Institute
Jeff Shuren, Food and Drug Administration
Dean Sittig, University of Texas Health Science Center at Houston

Randy Spratt, McKesson
James Walker, Geisinger Health System
David Woods, Ohio State University

We would also like to acknowledge and thank those who provided the
committee and staff with their insights during the report process:

Elisabeth Belmont, MaineHealth
Pamela Brewer, Healthcare Information and Management Systems
    Society
Mary Ann Chaffee, Surescripts
Sarah Corley, NextGen Healthcare Information Systems, Inc.
James B. Couch, Patient Safety Solutions, LLC
Carl Dvorak, Epic
Edward Fotsch, PDR Network
John Glaser, Siemens Healthcare
Ellen Harper, Cerner Corporation
Gay Johannes, Cerner Corporation
Bruce Leshine, LeClairRyan
Svetlana Lowry, National Institute of Standards and Technology (NIST)
Bakul Patel, Food and Drug Administration
Matt Quinn, NIST
Russell Roberson, GE
Mark Segal, GE
Matthew Wynia, American Medical Association
David Yakimischak, Surescripts

The committee would also like thank the following commissioned
paper authors:

Joan Ash, Oregon Health & Sciences University
Daniel Castro, Information Technology and Innovation Foundation
William Hersh, Oregon Health & Sciences University
Charles Kilo, Oregon Health & Sciences University
Hank Levine, Levine, Blaszak, Block & Boothby, LLP
Carmit McMullen, Kaiser Permanente Center for Health Research
Beth Rosenberg
Michael Shapiro, Oregon Health & Science University
Luke Stewart, Information Technology and Innovation Foundation
Joseph Wasserman, Oregon Health & Science University

In addition, there were many Institute of Medicine staff members who
helped throughout the study process. The staff would like to thank Patrick

Burke, Cassandra Cacace, Marton Cavani, Seth Glickman, Linda Kilroy, William McLeod, and Erin Wilhelm for their time and support to further the committee's efforts during the study process.

Finally, we would like to thank and recognize Jodi Daniel and Kathy Kenyon from the Office of the National Coordinator for Health IT for their support and the U.S. Department of Health and Human Services for sponsoring this study.

Contents

APPENDIXES

Abbreviations and Acronyms

ADE	adverse drug event
AHRQ	Agency for Healthcare Research and Quality
AMIA	American Medical Informatics Association
ASRS	Aviation Safety Reporting System
CCP	critical control point
CDS	clinical decision support
CIO	chief information officer
CMS	Centers for Medicare & Medicaid Services
CPOE	computerized provider order entry
EHR	electronic health record
EU	European Union
FAA	Federal Aviation Administration
FDA	Food and Drug Administration
HACCP	Hazard Analysis Critical Control Points
HFMEA®	Healthcare Failure Modes-and-Effects Analysis
HHS	U.S. Department of Health and Human Services
HIMSS	Healthcare Information and Management Systems Society
HIS	health information system
HITECH	Health Information Technology for Economic and Clinical Health
HL7	Health Level 7

ICU	intensive care unit
IOM	Institute of Medicine
ISO	International Organization for Standardization
IT	information technology
LOINC	Logical Observation Identifiers Names and Codes
NCCD	National Center for Cognitive Informatics and Decision Making in Healthcare
NCQA	National Committee for Quality Assurance
NIST	National Institute of Standards and Technology
NLM	National Library of Medicine
NQF	National Quality Forum
NRC	Nuclear Regulatory Commission
NTSB	National Transportation Safety Board
ONC	Office of the National Coordinator for Health Information Technology
ONC-ATCB	ONC-authorized testing and certification body
PCP	primary care physician
PHR	personal health record
PROMIS	problem-oriented medical information system
PSIP	Patient Safety through Intelligent Procedures in Medication
PSO	Patient Safety Organization
QSR	Quality System Regulation
SAFROS	Safety for Robotic Surgery
SNOMED	Systematized Nomenclature for Medicine
TURF	task, user, representation, and function
VA	U.S. Department of Veterans Affairs
WHO	World Health Organization

Summary

The Institute of Medicine (IOM) report *To Err Is Human* estimated that 44,000-98,000 lives are lost every year due to medical errors in hospitals and led to the widespread recognition that health care is not safe enough, catalyzing a revolution to improve the quality of care.[1] Despite considerable effort, patient safety has not yet improved to the degree hoped for in the IOM report *Crossing the Quality Chasm*. One strategy the nation has turned to for safer, more effective care is the widespread use of health information technologies (health IT).[2] The U.S. government is investing billions of dollars toward meaningful use of effective health IT so all Americans can benefit from the use of electronic health records (EHRs) by 2014.

Health IT is playing an ever-larger role in the care of patients, and some components of health IT have significantly improved the quality of health care and reduced medical errors. Continuing to use paper records can place patients at unnecessary risk for harm and substantially constrain the country's ability to reform health care. However, concerns about harm from the use of health IT have emerged. To protect America's health, health IT must be designed and used in ways that maximize patient safety while minimizing harm. Information technology can better help patients if it becomes more usable, more interoperable, and easier to implement and

---

[1] The IOM identified six aims of quality improvement, stating that health care should be safe, effective, patient-centered, timely, efficient, and equitable.

[2] Health IT can also be referred to as health information systems and health information and communications technology, among others. This report employs the term health IT but recognizes that these other, broader terms are also used.

1

maintain. This report explains the potential benefits and risks of health IT and asks for greater transparency, accountability, and reporting.

In this report, health IT includes a broad range of products, including EHRs,[3] patient engagement tools (e.g., personal health records [PHRs] and secure patient portals), and health information exchanges; excluded is software for medical devices. Clinicians expect health IT to support delivery of high-quality care in several ways, including storing comprehensive health data, providing clinical decision support, facilitating communication, and reducing medical errors. Health IT is not a single product; it encompasses a technical system of computers and software that operates in the context of a larger sociotechnical system—a collection of hardware and software working in concert within an organization that includes people, processes, and technology.

It is widely believed that health IT, when designed, implemented, and used appropriately, can be a positive enabler to transform the way care is delivered. Designed and applied inappropriately, health IT can add an additional layer of complexity to the already complex delivery of health care, which can lead to unintended adverse consequences, for example dosing errors, failure to detect fatal illnesses, and delayed treatment due to poor human–computer interactions or loss of data.

In recognition of the rapid adoption of health IT, the Office of the National Coordinator for Health Information Technology (ONC) asked the IOM to establish a committee to explore how private and public actors can maximize the safety of health IT–assisted care. The committee interpreted its charge as making health IT–assisted care *safer* so the nation is in a better position to realize the potential benefits of health IT.

EVALUATING THE CURRENT STATE OF PATIENT SAFETY AND HEALTH IT

The expectations for safer care may be higher in a health IT–enabled environment as compared to a paper-based environment because the opportunity to improve patient care is much greater. The evidence in the literature about the impact of health IT on patient safety, as opposed to quality, is mixed but shows that the challenges facing safer health care and safer use of health IT involve the people and clinical implementation as much as the technology. The literature describes significant improvements in some aspects of care in health care institutions with mature health IT. For example, the use of computerized prescribing and bar-coding systems has been shown

---

[3] "Electronic health records" is used as the desired term because it is more inclusive of the way electronic records are being used currently than "electronic medical records." EHRs include clinical decision support tools, computerized provider order entry systems, and e-prescribing systems.

to improve medication safety. But the generalizability of the literature across the health care system may be limited. While some studies suggest improvements in patient safety can be made, others have found no effect. Instances of health IT–associated harm have been reported. However, **little published evidence could be found quantifying the magnitude of the risk.**

Several reasons health IT–related safety data are lacking include the absence of measures and a central repository (or linkages among decentralized repositories) to collect, analyze, and act on information related to safety of this technology. Another impediment to gathering safety data is contractual barriers (e.g., nondisclosure, confidentiality clauses) that can prevent users from sharing information about health IT–related adverse events. These barriers limit users' abilities to share knowledge of risk-prone user interfaces, for instance through screenshots and descriptions of potentially unsafe processes. In addition, some vendors include language in their sales contracts and escape responsibility for errors or defects in their software (i.e., "hold-harmless clauses"). The committee believes these types of **contractual restrictions limit transparency, which significantly contributes to the gaps in knowledge of health IT–related patient safety risks.** These barriers to generating evidence pose unacceptable risks to safety.

EXAMINING THE CURRENT STATE OF THE ART IN SYSTEM SAFETY

Software-related safety issues are often ascribed to software coding errors or human errors in using the software. It is rarely that simple. Many problems with health IT relate to usability, implementation, and how software fits with clinical workflow. Focusing on coding or human errors often leads to neglect of other factors (e.g., usability, workflow, interoperability) that may increase the likelihood a patient safety event will occur. Furthermore, software—such as an EHR—is neither safe nor unsafe because safety of health IT cannot exist in isolation from its context of use. **Safety is an emergent property of a larger system that takes into account not just the software but also how it is used by clinicians.**

The larger system—often called a sociotechnical system—includes **technology** (e.g., software, hardware), **people** (e.g., clinicians, patients), **processes** (e.g., workflow), **organization** (e.g., capacity, decisions about how health IT is applied, incentives), and the **external environment** (e.g., regulations, public opinion). Adopting a sociotechnical perspective acknowledges that safety emerges from the interaction among various factors. Comprehensive safety analyses consider these factors taken as a whole and how they affect each other in an attempt to reduce the likelihood of an adverse event, rather than focusing on eliminating one "root cause" and ignoring other possible contributing factors.

OPPORTUNITIES TO BUILD SAFER SYSTEMS FOR HEALTH IT

Merely installing health IT in health care organizations will not result in improved care. Together, the design, implementation, and use of health IT affect its safe performance. **Safer implementation and use of health IT is a complex, dynamic process that requires a shared responsibility between vendors and health care organizations.**

Features of Safer Health IT

Safely functioning health IT should provide easy entry and retrieval of data, have simple and intuitive displays, and allow data to be easily transferred among health professionals. Many features of software contribute to its safe use, including usability and interoperability. Although definitive evidence is hard to produce, the committee believes **poor user-interface design, poor workflow, and complex data interfaces are threats to patient safety.**

Similarly, **lack of system interoperability is a barrier to improving clinical decisions and patient safety,** as it can limit data available for clinical decision making. Laboratory data have been relatively easy to exchange because good standards exist such as Logical Observation Identifiers Names and Codes (LOINC) and are widely accepted. However, important information such as problem lists and medication lists are not easily transmitted and understood by the receiving health IT product because existing standards have not been uniformly adopted. Interoperability must extend throughout the continuum of care; standards need to be developed and implemented to support interaction between health IT products that contain disparate data.

Opportunities to Improve the Design and Development of Technologies

Application of quality management practices needs to be a high priority for design and development activities. Creating safer systems begins with user-centered design principles and continues with adequate testing and quality assessments conducted in actual and/or simulated clinical environments. Vendors should not only create useful functions in their software but also understand how user-interface design affects the clinical setting and workflow where the applications are to be used, as well as support for activities within a health professional's scope of practice.

Opportunities to Improve Safety in the Use of Health IT

Safety considerations need to be embedded throughout the implementation process, including the stages of planning and goal setting, deployment, stabilization, optimization, and transformation. Selecting the right software requires a comprehensive understanding of the data and information needs of the organization and the capabilities of the system. Vendors take primary responsibility for the design and development of technologies, ideally with iterative feedback from users. Users assume responsibility for safe implementation and work with vendors throughout the health IT implementation process. The partnership to develop, implement, and optimize systems is a shared responsibility where vendors and users help each other achieve the safest possible applications of health IT.

It is important to recognize that health IT products generally cannot be installed out of the box. Users need to customize products judiciously to appropriately match their needs and capabilities—in both functionality and complexity of operation. The process of implementing software is critical to optimizing value and mitigating patient safety risks. **A constant, ongoing commitment to safety—from acquisition to implementation and maintenance—is needed to achieve safer, more effective care.** Testing at each of these stages is needed to ensure successful use of health IT.

Responsible use requires diligent surveillance for evolving needs, gaps, performance issues, and mismatches between user needs and system performance, unsafe conditions, and adverse events. The committee believes certain actions are required by private and public entities to monitor safety in order to protect the public's health and provides the following recommendations to improve health IT safety nationwide—optimizing their use to achieve national health goals, while reducing the risks of their use resulting in inadvertent harm.

> **Recommendation 1: The Secretary of Health and Human Services (HHS) should publish an action and surveillance plan within 12 months that includes a schedule for working with the private sector to assess the impact of health IT on patient safety and minimizing the risk of its implementation and use. The plan should specify:**
>   a. **The Agency for Healthcare Research and Quality (AHRQ) and the National Library of Medicine (NLM) should expand their funding of research, training, and education of safe practices as appropriate, including measures specifically related to the design, implementation, usability, and safe use of health IT by all users, including patients.**
>   b. **The Office of the National Coordinator for Health Information Technology should expand its funding of processes that promote safety that should be followed in the development of health IT products, including standardized testing procedures to be used by manufacturers and health care organizations to assess the safety of health IT products.**

   c. The ONC and AHRQ should work with health IT vendors and health care organizations to promote postdeployment safety testing of EHRs for high-prevalence, high-impact EHR-related patient safety risks.

   d. Health care accrediting organizations should adopt criteria relating to EHR safety.

   e. AHRQ should fund the development of new methods for measuring the impact of health IT on safety using data from EHRs.

PATIENTS' AND FAMILIES' USE OF HEALTH IT: CONCERNS ABOUT SAFETY

Health IT products are also being developed to engage and support patients and their families in decision making and management of their own personal health information. Examples of electronic patient engagement tools include PHRs (both integrated and freestanding), mobile applications, and tools for assessing day-to-day health status (e.g., weight loss), and continue to evolve rapidly. The increasing use of health IT by consumers, patients, and families creates an urgent need for the development and support of a research agenda for these tools.

A SHARED RESPONSIBILITY FOR IMPROVING HEALTH IT SAFETY

Health IT safety is contingent on how the technology is designed, implemented, used, and fits into clinical workflow, requiring the cooperation of both vendors and users. In the absence of a single accountable party, policy makers need to act on behalf of the public good to promote and monitor health IT safety. The committee believes this is best accomplished through collaboration between the private and public sectors.

The private sector must play a major role in making health IT safer, but it will need support from and close collaboration with the public sector. Currently, there is no systematic regulation or sense of shared accountability for product functioning, liability is shifted primarily onto users, and there is no way to publicly track adverse outcomes. Therefore, when instances that either cause or could result in harm occur, there is no authority to collect, analyze, and disseminate learning. Lack of sufficient vendor action to build safer products, or regulatory requirements to do so, threatens patient safety. Access to details of patient safety risks is essential to a properly functioning market where users identify the product that best suits their needs. Users need to share information about risks and adverse events with other users and vendors. Legal clauses shifting liability from vendors to users discourage sharing.

Recommendation 2: The Secretary of HHS should ensure insofar as possible that health IT vendors support the free exchange of information about health IT experiences and issues and not prohibit sharing of such information, including details (e.g., screenshots) relating to patient safety.

Once information about patient safety risks is available, comparative user experiences can be shared. Currently, users cannot communicate effectively their experiences with health IT. In other industries, product reviews are available where users can rate their experiences with products and share lessons learned. A consumer guide for health IT safety could help identify safety concerns, increasing system transparency.

To gather objective information about health IT products, researchers should have access to both test versions of software provided by vendors and software already integrated in user organizations. Users should be able to compare and share their experiences and other measures of safety from health IT products.

Recommendation 3: The ONC should work with the private and public sectors to make comparative user experiences across vendors publicly available.

Another area necessary for making health IT safer is the development of measures. Inasmuch as the committee's charge is to recommend policies and practices that lead to *safer* use of health IT, the nation needs reliable means of assessing the current state and monitoring for improvement. Currently, no entity is developing such measures; Recommendation 1 is for AHRQ, the NLM, and the ONC to fund development of these measures. The lack of measures and diversity of involved parties suggests a coordinating body is needed to oversee the development, application, and evaluation of measures of safety of health IT use. Best practices will need to ensure health IT is developed and implemented with safety as a priority.

Recommendation 4: The Secretary of HHS should fund a new Health IT Safety Council to evaluate criteria for assessing and monitoring the safe use of health IT and the use of health IT to enhance safety. This council should operate within an existing voluntary consensus standards organization.

This function could be housed within existing organizations, such as the National Quality Forum.

Because threats to health IT safety can arise before, during, and after implementation, it is also useful to design methods to monitor health IT safety. Standards development organizations such as the American National Standards Institute and the Association for the Advancement of Medical Instrumentation could seek input from a broad group of stakeholders when developing these standards, criteria, and tests. Additionally, vendor attestation that they have addressed specific safety issues in the design and development of their products can be important. Best practices for acquisition and implementation of health IT need to be developed. Development of postimplementation tests would help users monitor whether their systems meet certain safety benchmarks. Applying these tests is also a way for users to work with vendors to ensure that products have been installed correctly; accreditation organizations, such as The Joint Commission, could require conduct of these safety tests as part of their accreditation criteria.

Finally, the committee found **successful adoption of change requires education and training of the workforce.** Basic levels of competence, knowledge, and skill are needed to navigate the highly complex implementation of health IT. Because health IT exists at the intersection of multiple disciplines, a variety of professionals will need training in a number of established disciplines such as health systems, IT, and clinical care.

The Role of the Public Sector: Strategic Guidance and Oversight

A shared learning environment should be fostered to the fullest extent possible by the private sector, but, in some instances, the government needs to provide guidance and direction to private-sector efforts and to correct misaligned market forces. An appropriate balance must be reached between government oversight and market innovation. To encourage innovation and shared learning environments, the committee adopted the following general principles for government oversight:

- Focus on shared learning,
- Maximize transparency,
- Be nonpunitive,
- Identify appropriate levels of accountability, and
- Minimize burden.

The committee believes HHS should take the following actions to improve health IT safety.

First, to improve transparency and safety, it is necessary to identify the products being used and to whom any actions need to be directed. Having a mechanism to accomplish this is important so that when new knowledge about safety or performance arises, other users and products that could also be vulnerable can be identified. The ONC employed a similar mechanism for EHR vendors to list their products in implementing the meaningful use program. The committee supports continuation of the ONC's efforts to list all products certified for meaningful use in a single database as a first step for ensuring safety.

> **Recommendation 5: All health IT vendors should be required to publicly register and list their products with the ONC, initially beginning with EHRs certified for the meaningful use program.**

Second, by establishing quality management principles and processes in health IT, vendors can improve the safety of their product lines. Experiences from other industries suggest the best approach to proactively creating highly reliable products is not to certify each individual product but to make sure organizations have adopted quality management principles and processes in the design and development of products.

While many vendors already have some types of quality management principles and processes in place, not all vendors do and to what standard they are held is unknown. An industry standard is needed to ensure comprehensive industry adoption. To this end, the committee believes adoption of quality management principles and processes should be mandatory for all health IT vendors. The ONC, Food and Drug Administration (FDA), and health IT certification bodies are examples of organizations that could potentially administer this function.

> **Recommendation 6: The Secretary of HHS should specify the quality and risk management process requirements that health IT vendors must adopt, with a particular focus on human factors, safety culture, and usability.**

Third, to quantify patient safety risks, reports of adverse events need to be collected, supplementing private-sector efforts. High-priority health IT–related adverse events include death, serious injury, and unsafe conditions. Analyses of unsafe conditions would produce important information that could have a great impact on improving patient safety and enable adoption of corrective actions that could prevent death or serious injury.

Regular reporting of adverse events is widely used to identify and rectify vulnerabilities that threaten safety for the purposes of learning. However, learning about safety of health IT is limited because there are currently no comprehensive analyses available about health IT–related adverse events, no consequences for failing to discover and report evidence about harm, and no aggregation of data for learning. In other countries and industries, reporting systems all differ with respect to their design, but the majority employ **reporting that is voluntary, confidential, and nonpunitive.** Creating a nonpunitive environment is essential for the success of voluntary reporting systems. Reports must be collected for the purpose of learning and should not be used to address accountability.

The committee believes reports of health IT–related adverse events and unsafe conditions that are verified and free of user-identifying information should be transparently available to the public. The committee believes reporting of deaths, serious injuries, or unsafe conditions should be mandatory for vendors. Direction will need to come from a federal entity with adequate expertise, capacity, and authority to act on reports of health IT–related adverse events. The Secretary of HHS should designate an entity and provide it with the necessary resources to do so.

Current user reporting efforts are generally not coordinated with one another and not collected in a systematic manner; a more streamlined reporting system is needed. AHRQ has developed a common format that precisely defines the components of a field report for health IT–related adverse events or risks. Reports by users should remain voluntary and the identities of reporters should not be discoverable under any circumstance. Patient Safety Organizations are examples of entities that can protect this information from discovery. User-reported health IT–related adverse events should be collected by a central repository and also be sent to the appropriate vendor.

> **Recommendation 7: The Secretary of HHS should establish a mechanism for both vendors and users to report health IT–related deaths, serious injuries, or unsafe conditions.**
> a. Reporting of health IT–related adverse events should be mandatory for vendors.
> b. Reporting of health IT–related adverse events by users should be voluntary, confidential, and nonpunitive.
> c. Efforts to encourage reporting should be developed, such as removing the perceptual, cultural, contractual, legal, and logistical barriers to reporting.

However, reports of patient safety incidents are only one part of a larger solution to maximize the safety of health IT–assisted care. **The power to improve safety lies not just with reporting requirements, but with the ability to act on and learn from reports.** To this end, two distinct functions are also needed: (1) aggregating and analyzing reports and (2) investigating the circumstances associated with safety incidents to determine the conditions that contribute to those incidents. Through these processes, lessons learned can be developed so similar incidents will be less likely to occur in the future. To maximize the effectiveness of reports, the collection, aggregation and analysis, and investigation of reports should be coupled as closely as possible.

Ideally, all reports of health IT–related adverse events would be aggregated and analyzed by a single entity that would identify reports for immediate investigation. Reports to this entity have to include identifiable data to allow investigators to follow up in the event the reported incident requires investigation. The entity would investigate two categories of reports: (1) reports that result in death or serious injury and (2) reports of unsafe conditions. Prioritization among the reports should be determined on a risk-based hazard analysis. In keeping with the principle of transparency, reports and results of investigations should be made public. A feedback loop from the investigatory entity back to both vendors and users is essential to allow groups to rectify systemic issues found that introduce risk.

The committee considered a number of potential organizations that could objectively analyze reports of unsafe conditions, as well as conduct investigations into health IT–related adverse events in the way the committee envisions, including FDA, the ONC, AHRQ, and the private sector. The committee concluded that investigating patient safety incidents does not match the internal expertise of any existing entity, as the needed functions are under the jurisdiction of multiple federal agencies and efforts are generally uncoordinated and not comprehensive.

The committee believes development of an independent, federal entity could perform the needed analytic and investigative functions in a transparent, nonpunitive manner. It would be similar in structure to the National Transportation Safety Board, an independent federal agency created by Congress to conduct safety investigations. The entity would make nonbinding recommendations to the Secretary of HHS. Nonbinding recommendations provide flexibility, allowing the Secretary, health care organizations, vendors, and external experts to collectively determine the best course forward. Because current federal agencies do not have this as their charge, nor the baseline funding to take on these activities, the committee believes an independent, federal entity is the best option to provide a platform to support shared learning at a national level.

Recommendation 8: The Secretary of HHS should recommend that Congress establish an independent federal entity for investigating patient safety deaths, serious injuries, or potentially unsafe conditions associated with health IT. This entity should also monitor and analyze data and publicly report results of these activities.

When combined, removing contractual restrictions, promoting public reporting, and having a system in place for independent investigations can be a powerful force for improving patient safety.

Next Steps

Achieving transparency and safer health IT products and safer use of health IT will require the cooperation of all stakeholders. Without more information about the magnitude and types of harm, other mechanisms will be necessary to motivate the market to correct itself. The committee offers a two-stage approach, with its recommended actions as the first stage to provide a better understanding of the threats to patient safety.

The current state of safety and health IT is not acceptable; specific actions are required to improve the safety of health IT. The first eight recommendations are intended to create conditions and incentives to encourage substantial industry-driven change without formal regulation. However, because the private sector to date has not taken sufficient action on its own, the committee believes a follow-up recommendation is needed to formally regulate health IT.[4] If the actions recommended to the private and public sectors are not effective as determined by the Secretary of HHS, the Secretary should direct FDA to exercise all authorities to regulate health IT.

The committee was of mixed opinion on how FDA regulation would impact the pace of innovation by industry but identified several areas of concern regarding immediate FDA regulation. The current FDA framework is oriented toward conventional, out-of-the-box, turnkey devices. However, health IT has multiple different characteristics, suggesting that a more flexible regulatory framework will be needed in this area to achieve the goals of product quality and safety without unduly constraining market innovation. For example, as a software-based product, health IT has a product life cycle very different from that of conventional technologies. These products exhibit great diversity in features, functions, and scope of intended and actual use, which tend to evolve over the life of the product. Taking a phased, risk-based approach can help address this concern. FDA has chosen to not exercise regulatory authority over EHRs, and controversy exists over whether some health IT products such as EHRs should be considered medical devices. If the Secretary deems it necessary for FDA to regulate EHRs and other currently nonregulated health IT products, clear determinations will need to be made about whether all health IT products classify as medical devices for the purposes of regulation. If FDA regulation is deemed necessary, FDA will need to commit sufficient resources and add capacity and expertise to be effective.

The Secretary should report annually to Congress and the public on the progress of efforts to improve the safety of health IT, beginning 12 months from the release of this report. In these reports, the Secretary should make

---

[4] One member disagrees with the committee and would immediately regulate health IT as a Class III medical device, as outlined in Appendix E.

clear the reasons why further oversight actions are or are not needed. In parallel, the Secretary should ask FDA to begin planning the framework needed for potential regulation consistent with Recommendations 1 through 8 so that, if she deems FDA regulation to be necessary, the agency will be ready to act, allowing for the protection of patient safety without further delay. The committee recognizes that not all of its recommendations can be acted on by the Secretary alone and that some will require congressional action.

> Recommendation 9a: The Secretary of HHS should monitor and publicly report on the progress of health IT safety annually beginning in 2012. If progress toward safety and reliability is not sufficient as determined by the Secretary, the Secretary should direct FDA to exercise all available authorities to regulate EHRs, health information exchanges, and PHRs.

> Recommendation 9b: The Secretary should immediately direct FDA to begin developing the necessary framework for regulation. Such a framework should be in place if and when the Secretary decides the state of health IT safety requires FDA regulation as stipulated in Recommendation 9a above.

FUTURE RESEARCH FOR CARE TRANSFORMATION

The committee identified a number of research gaps during its information gathering. Research is needed to continue to build the evidence to determine how to develop and adopt safer health IT most effectively. A greater body of conclusive research is needed to fully meet the potential of health IT for ensuring patient safety.

> Recommendation 10: HHS, in collaboration with other research groups, should support cross-disciplinary research toward the use of health IT as part of a learning health care system. Products of this research should be used to inform the design, testing, and use of health IT. Specific areas of research include
>   a. User-centered design and human factors applied to health IT,
>   b. Safe implementation and use of health IT by all users,
>   c. Sociotechnical systems associated with health IT, and
>   d. Impact of policy decisions on health IT use in clinical practice.

Creating an infrastructure that supports learning about and improving the safety of health IT is needed to achieve better health care. Proactive steps must be taken to ensure that health IT is developed and implemented with safety as a primary focus through the development of industry-wide measures, standards, and criteria for safety. Surveillance mechanisms are needed to identify, capture, and investigate adverse events to continually improve the safety of health IT. Transparency and cooperation between the private and public sectors are critical to creating the necessary infrastructure to build safer systems that will lead to better care for all Americans.

1

Introduction

"To Err Is Human"
"Crossing the Quality Chasm"

Together, the above phrases—titles of reports—catalyzed a revolution in American health care to ensure patient safety and improve quality of care. *To Err Is Human* estimated that 44,000-98,000 lives are lost in hospitals every year due to medical errors and led to the widespread recognition that health care is not as safe as it should be (IOM, 1999). With an emphasis on improving quality,[1] better results were thought to be achievable (IOM, 2001).

Subsequent research further documented the deficiencies in the quality and safety of American health care. Early work found evidence-based practice is only followed 55 percent of the time (McGlynn et al., 2003), and ensuing studies have reconfirmed that medical errors continue to be prevalent, as more than 1.5 million preventable adverse drug events occur annually (IOM, 2006). Adverse events can result from almost any type of interaction with the care system, at any point during care delivery, and in all care settings. Events can be the result of human, technological, and systems errors and can be classified as errors of commission (a direct consequence of treatment) or errors of omission (failure to undertake an action that should have been completed). Specific to safety, there has been a tendency to assume that a focus on quality will of necessity result in improved safety.

---

[1] The Institute of Medicine (IOM) identified six aims of quality improvement, stating that health care should be safe, effective, patient-centered, timely, efficient, and equitable (2001).

This assumption may have delayed awareness of the need for a robust framework focused on safety alone.

Perhaps more important, these studies brought to light the critical concept of systemness, which recognizes that health care is a collection of disparate fragmented parts with many individual actors, each seeking to do their best by the patient instead of health professionals within a comprehensive "system." This lack of systems to improve coordination in part fostered the promulgation of poor-quality, unsafe health care. Although the attention to systems of care have increased greatly, many of the efforts in the 10 years since *To Err Is Human* and *Crossing the Quality Chasm* have focused on processes of care as a first step, with the end goal of creating a comprehensive system of high-quality and safe care. These studies and those in the next section focused on quality and safety in health care overall. This background is needed to understand the context for discussing patient safety related to health information technology (health IT).[2]

PATIENT SAFETY

More than 10 years since these landmark patient safety reports, there is considerable controversy about how much improvement in safety has actually occurred. Clearly some progress has been made with respect to specific processes, such as high rates of prescribing beta-blockers at discharge to patients presenting with an acute myocardial infarction (Chassin et al., 2010), and significantly reduced surgical mortality rates (Neily et al., 2010). Nationwide efforts were undertaken to reduce the number of medical errors in all care settings, and campaigns were developed to increase awareness, reduce risk factors, and develop a framework for high-quality care.

Despite these efforts, quality improvement throughout much of the U.S. health care system is still proceeding at a glacial pace. The *National Healthcare Quality Report* by the Agency for Healthcare Research and Quality (AHRQ) revealed that while nearly two-thirds of 179 measures of health care quality did show improvement, the median annual rate of change was only 2.3 percent. Several quality measures relating to cancer screening and diabetes management actually worsened during this time (AHRQ, 2010).

In terms of safety, several new studies have recently been published sug-

---

[2] Health IT is a term that is used somewhat interchangeably with other terms such as health information systems, health information and communications technology, and informatics. The terms are not necessarily defined the same way; for example, informatics—defined as a scientific field that draws upon the information sciences and related technology to enhance the use of the knowledge base of the health sciences to improve the health of individuals and populations through care, basic biomedical and clinical research, education, management, and policy—is a broader field than health IT. This report employs the term health IT but recognizes these other, broader terms are also used.

gesting that patients continued to experience high rates of safety problems during hospital stays. Indeed, one study found adverse events continue to occur in as many as one-third of hospital patients (Classen et al., 2011). These adverse events occur in hospitalized patients even in regions where there has been a heavy programmatic focus on improving patient safety in hospitals (Landrigan et al., 2010). Safety problems also plague Medicare beneficiaries—a study suggests that more than 27 percent of Medicare beneficiaries will experience an adverse event during their hospitalizations, with half of these patients suffering more severe adverse events (HHS, 2010a).

These patient safety problems are not just limited to inpatient care. *To Err Is Human* recognized that more patients could be harmed by errors in ambulatory settings because more medical care is delivered outside of hospitals than inside. A recent review of malpractice claims concluded that 52 percent of all paid malpractice claims for all physician services involved ambulatory services, and almost two-thirds of these claims involved a major injury or death (Bishop et al., 2011).

Important differences exist between the inpatient and ambulatory settings regarding patient safety, including the types of errors seen (IOM, 1999), the relative importance of patient responsibility for following through on care decisions, and the different organizational and regulatory structures in place (Gandhi and Lee, 2010). As a result, it cannot be assumed that interventions to improve hospital safety will be applicable in the ambulatory setting, which deserves focused attention of its own. In recognition of this, an expert consensus conference to establish an agenda for research in ambulatory patient safety recognized that knowledge of ambulatory patient safety was lacking (Hammons et al., 2001). A recent 10-year review of ambulatory patient safety literature concluded that some progress has been made in understanding ambulatory safety, major gaps remain, and virtually no experiments or demonstrations have been done that show how to improve it (Lorincz et al., 2011).

This new refocus on patient safety as a specific system priority is best exemplified by a new Department of Health and Human Services (HHS) initiative with a sole focus on patient safety. Policy makers have recently recognized the significant challenges in improving patient safety across the continuum of care and the lack of progress over the past decade. HHS recently announced a national initiative called the Partnership for Patients, aimed at reducing preventable hospital-acquired conditions and complications, that would result in about 1.8 million fewer injuries to patients and would save more than 60,000 lives over 3 years. The partnership also aims to reduce preventable complications during care transitions, thereby cutting hospital readmissions by 20 percent from 2010 levels (HHS, 2011). This may herald a new national focus on patient safety over the next decade in the United States.

As these findings indicate, the opportunity to continue to improve is great, with many tools yet to be developed and effectively implemented. In virtually every report on patient safety summarized above, health IT has been identified as a critical tool to both measure and improve patient safety. Yet despite the possibility that health IT can enhance the safety and effectiveness of care, the widespread adoption and safe use of health IT products is still relatively immature. Technical and organizational limitations exist that can make health IT difficult to use effectively to improve the safety and quality of care.

HEALTH IT

For the purposes of this report, health IT includes a broad range of products, including electronic health records (EHRs),[3] patient engagement tools (e.g., personal health records), and health information exchanges; excluded is software for medical devices (e.g., software in an implantable cardioverter-defibrillator). The use of data support systems in health settings began as administrative tools to facilitate billing processes and other related transactions. More recently, health IT has evolved to EHRs and other forms of technology that engage not just in transactions and data storage but also decision support and the capacity for clinicians and patients to see the patient's clinical progress and data more easily. Clinicians and health care systems can potentially benefit from studying populations of similar patients, leading to learning health care systems. Clinicians expect health IT to support delivery of high-quality care in several ways, including storing comprehensive health data, providing clinical decision support, facilitating communication, engaging patients, and reducing medical errors. In the near future, it is likely that patients, particularly those with chronic illnesses, will consistently use the Internet to track their own health through personal health records and handheld device applications. Current health IT products are still improving their capacity to increase communications and reduce errors by making the right thing to do easier to do. It is important that health IT maximize patient safety while minimizing harm.

Adoption of health IT has been slow and is not yet widespread in the United States. Although adoption rates have increased significantly over the past decade, only 50.7 percent of office-based physicians use any type of EHR, with 10.1 percent reporting use of a fully functional record (Hsiao et al., 2010) (see Figure 1-1).

---

[3] In this report, electronic health record will be used as the desired term over electronic medical record because it is more inclusive of the way electronic records are being used currently. EHRs include clinical decision support tools, computerized provider order entry systems, and e-prescribing systems.

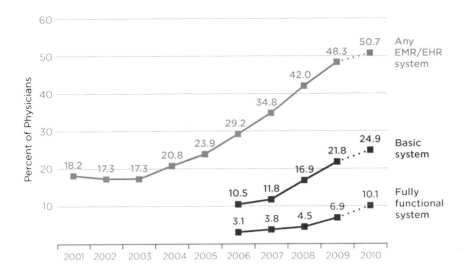

FIGURE 1-1
Percentage of office-based physicians with electronic medical records/electronic health records: United States, 2001–2009 and preliminary 2010.

NOTES: Any EMR/EHR is a medical or health record system that is either all or partially electronic (excluding systems solely for billing). The 2010 data are preliminary estimates (as show by dotted lines), based only on the mail survey. Estimates through 2009 include additional physicians sampled from community health centers; prior 2008 combined estimates were revised to include those physicians (4). Estimates of basic and fully functional systems prior to 2006 could not be computed because some items were not collected in the survey. Fully functional systems are a subset of basic systems. Some of the increase in fully functional systems between 2009 and 2010 may be related to a change in survey instruments and definitions of fully functional systems between 2009 and 2010. Includes nonfederal, office-based physicians. Excludes radiologists, anesthesiologists, and pathologists.

SOURCE: Hsiao et al. (2010); CDC/NCHS, National Ambulatory Medical Care Survey.

With respect to hospitals, 11.9 percent of U.S. hospitals use comprehensive EHRs (Jha et al., 2010). Many barriers to adopting health IT exist, including the complexity of training needed to integrate systems into new patterns and clinical workflows, the cost of acquiring and maintaining health IT, and the lack of resources to overcome barriers to implementation. As a result, the current culture of care delivery is often not ready for widespread safer and more effective use of health IT.

In contrast to the United States, other countries have achieved much higher adoption rates of EHRs. Denmark has had fully electronic patient records for 10 years, and countries such as the Netherlands, Australia,

Singapore, and Canada also are much further along than the United States (see Chapter 2). These countries report both efficiencies in operation and reductions in prescription error rates. Problems associated with health IT reported overseas, most recently highlighted in the United Kingdom's decision to end its National Programme for IT after spending £6.4 of the £11 billion allotted for the program, reflect complex issues of contracts, product capabilities, and vendor performance, not necessarily patient safety (Whalen, 2011).

A report by the President's Council of Advisers on Science and Technology concluded that the full potential of health IT to improve the quality and cost of health care has not yet been realized. Many advances will be needed, from lifting barriers (e.g., eliminating the proprietary nature of products to promote interoperability, broadening the ways in which data are used, ensuring privacy and security) to more innovative and competitive health IT products (PCAST, 2010).

In an effort to improve health care, the U.S. government has invested and will continue to invest billions of dollars toward the meaningful use of effective health IT in the hopes of improving the quality of care, decreasing the cost of care through improved efficiency, and guiding clinicians to choose the most effective care interventions. In 2004, the Office of the National Coordinator for Health Information Technology (ONC) was established by executive order within the Office of the Secretary of HHS. It was created in statute by the Health Information Technology for Economic and Clinical Health (HITECH) Act, part of the American Recovery and Reinvestment Act of 2009. Working toward the goal of bringing EHRs to all Americans by 2014, the mission of the ONC is to both coordinate development of a national health IT infrastructure and support and promote meaningful use of EHRs. The ONC is supported directly and indirectly by several federal advisory bodies (ONC, 2011). Those directly involved include the following:

- The Health IT Policy Committee was provided for in the HITECH Act to make recommendations to the National Coordinator for Health IT toward development of a policy framework for a nationwide health information infrastructure.
- The Health IT Standards Committee was established at the same time as the Policy Committee for the purpose of making recommendations regarding standards and certification criteria for the electronic exchange and use of health IT to the National Coordinator.
- The National Committee on Vital and Health Statistics was established in 1949 to advise the Secretary of HHS in issues related to health data, statistics, and national information policy. Its National

Health Information Infrastructure report created the vision for the emerging system (NCVHS, 2001).

Indirectly, the ONC receives helpful advice from a number of groups, including the advisory groups for the National Library of Medicine, AHRQ, multiple Boards of Scientific Counselors of the Centers for Disease Control and Prevention, the Visiting Committee on Advanced Technology of the National Institute for Standards and Technology, and the multiple advisory committees of the Food and Drug Administration.

In collaboration with many private efforts and other public agencies, these groups have been instrumental in advancing the development of an initial framework for health IT. Although these efforts have been essential to advancing the state of health IT, much more work is needed before all Americans will have access to health IT–assisted care.

Development of health IT–assisted care is also being encouraged by the broader health policy environment. Safe, interoperable health IT is a foundational component of strategies such as accountable care organizations and the patient-centered medical home. The promise of these movements to reduce costs and improve patient outcomes assumes that high-quality patient data can be shared reliably and effectively among providers. These movements, among others, are likely to influence the speed of adoption and broaden the functions of health IT considerably (NCVHS, 2001). In contrast to these possible future uses, it is clear that current health IT implementations are often complex, cumbersome, and brittle in ways that may also have negative effects on clinician performance (AHRQ, 2009; HIMSS, 2009; PCAST, 2010).

INTERSECTION OF PATIENT SAFETY AND HEALTH IT

Health IT is not one specific product that, once implemented, can automatically result in highly safe and effective health care. It encompasses a technical system of computers, software, and devices that operate in the context of a larger sociotechnical system—a collection of hardware and software working in concert within an organization that includes people, processes, and workflow. It is widely believed that, when designed and used appropriately, health IT can help create an ecosystem of safer care while also producing a variety of benefits such as reductions in administrative costs, improved clinical performance, and better communication between patients and caregivers. In this view, it can be a positive, transformative force for delivering health care. However, the assumption that the aforementioned benefits are highly correlated with health IT has not been adequately tested, and there are some indications that the features needed to acquire one benefit may actually frustrate efforts to achieve another.

In particular, there is a growing concern that health IT designs that maximize the potential for administrative and economic benefit may be creating new paths to failure. Reports of health IT becoming a distraction or cause of miscommunication raise the possibility that health IT may cause harm if it is poorly designed, implemented, or applied. Poorly designed, implemented, or applied, health IT can create new hazards in the already complex delivery of health care, requiring health care professionals to work around brittle software, adding steps needed to accomplish tasks, or presenting data in a nonintuitive format that can introduce risks that may lead to harm. Risks to patient safety also arise as a result of great heterogeneity in health IT products. As health IT products have become more intimately involved in the delivery of care, the potential for health IT–induced medical error, harm, or death has increased significantly. Examples of health IT–induced harm that can result in serious injury and death include dosing errors, failing to detect fatal illnesses, and delaying treatment due to poor human–computer interactions or loss of data (Aleccia, 2011; Associated Press, 2009; Graham and Dizikes, 2011; Schulte and Schwartz, 2010; Silver and Hamill, 2011; U.S. News, 2011).

The portfolio of research on health IT has included little regarding the general impact of health IT on safety of clinical care. The evidence in the literature about the impact of health IT on patient safety is mixed but shows that the challenges facing safer health care and safer use of health IT involve the people and clinical implementation as much as the technology. The literature does reflect improvements in some areas in well-established health care institutions, notably medication administration through use of computerized prescribing and bar-coding systems. But the evidence of health IT's impact on patient safety beyond medication safety and across the health care system is lacking. Although evidence suggests improvements in safety can be made, some studies have found health IT to have no effect on patient safety, and case reports such as those cited above show that it can also contribute to harm.

Advanced technology can create some new paths to failure at the same time that it blocks others. These new forms of failure are often hard to anticipate and may go unnoticed or be misidentified until the introduction of the new technology is well advanced. The resulting shift in the locus of failure can make the evaluation of the impact of technology on safety difficult, especially if the contribution of technology to the new forms of failure is not appreciated (Woods et al., 2010). Given the large investments being made in health IT, there is a great need to ensure that the new technology is actually improving safety of care.

IOM COMMITTEE

The ONC's Health IT Policy Committee held a hearing on patient safety and health IT in February 2010 and recommended the ONC "commission a formal study to thoroughly evaluate health IT patient safety concerns, and to recommend additional actions and strategies to address those concerns" (HHS, 2010b). In September 2010, the ONC asked the Institute of Medicine (IOM) to make recommendations about how public and private actors can maximize the safety of health IT–assisted care (see Box 1-1). In response, the IOM established the Committee on Patient Safety and Health Information Technology.

The committee's report comes at a point in time characterized by a number of rather dramatic changes relating to health care in addition to major national health insurance and financial reforms. First, the HITECH legislation provides substantial incentives to accelerate the adoption of EHR systems. Second, there is an ongoing movement away from the historical

---

BOX 1-1
Statement of Task

An ad hoc committee will review the available evidence and the experience from the field on how the use of health information technology affects the safety of patient care and will make recommendations concerning how public and private actors can maximize the safety of health IT-assisted health care services. The committee will produce a report that will be both comprehensive and specific in terms of recommended options and opportunities for public and private interventions that may improve the safety of care that incorporates the use of electronic health records (EHRs) and other forms of health IT.

"Health IT-assisted care" means health care and services that incorporate and take advantage of health information technologies and health information exchange for the purpose of improving the processes and outcomes of health care services. Health IT-assisted care includes care supported by and involving EHRs, clinical decision support, computerized provider order entry, health information exchange, patient engagement technologies, and other health information technology used in clinical care.

The committee will (1) summarize existing knowledge of the effects of health IT on patient safety; (2) make recommendations to HHS regarding specific actions that federal agencies should take to maximize the safety of health IT-assisted care; and (3) make recommendations concerning how private actors can promote the safety of health IT-assisted care, and how the federal government can assist private actors in this regard.

model of physician autonomy to one focused on adherence to evidence-based guidelines and best practices that promote safe, high-quality care. Finally, the practice of medicine is inexorably moving from being based primarily upon knowledge of organs and organ systems to being based upon genomics and proteomics, which has major implications for data management capabilities. The aggregate impact of these tectonic shifts beneath health care and its related technologies and treatments is one that requires development of more complex yet reliable systems to assure high performance in the midst of great baseline challenges to achieving excellent outcomes.

Scope

In his statement to the committee, David Blumenthal, the then–National Coordinator, asked the committee to consider the full range of activities available in developing recommendations to assure the safety of health IT–assisted care (Blumenthal, 2010). The statement of task defines health IT very broadly and includes multiple types of technologies used in the delivery of health care services. The committee considered all stakeholders as having important roles in improving patient safety with respect to health IT. This includes patients and their families, health professionals, health care delivery organizations (ranging from small physician offices to large hospital systems), health IT vendors, accrediting agencies, professional societies, insurance companies, and the government.

Controversy exists regarding the impact of both the introduction of health IT and the use of health IT on patient safety. Proponents argue that published literature from trials generally support the claim that health IT can reduce particular types of failure, improve quality and safety, and reduce costs. Critics point to reports of health IT failures. This report does not attempt to resolve the controversy; instead it seeks to assess some of the important issues surrounding health IT and its introduction and to indicate the activities most likely to bring the potential value of health IT to the U.S. health care system. Therefore, while the committee recognizes that both risks and benefits are associated with health IT, it interpreted its charge as making health IT–assisted care *safer* so that the nation is in a better position to realize the potential benefits of health IT.

The committee did not examine a number of issues related to health IT, including whether health IT should be implemented, access to health IT products, medical liability, privacy, security, and standards. These are critical for the ONC to address in order to achieve its mission of having widespread use of EHRs by 2014. Similarly, the validity and use of information from common Internet sites applied to specific patient situations during delivery of care is also important in the changing health care delivery environment but was not considered in the scope of this report. The committee also did not consider recommendations to address the broader issues associated with health care safety. This report focuses on patient safety as it relates to health IT and the delivery of care and will therefore concentrate on the aspects of health IT directly pertaining to safety.

Methods

To address the statement of task, the committee conducted a wide-ranging evaluation of the literature to gather evidence about patient safety and health IT (see Appendix B) and received input in a variety of forums. Over the course of this 12-month study, the committee met in person three times. The committee also benefited by engaging with the public during two workshops where it received statements from various stakeholder organizations. Additionally, the committee solicited input from the public and specifically the EHR vendor community.[4] Public comments included both statements about how a health IT product had improved the safety of an organization as well as instances of harm. Vendors described various processes adopted to both receive and handle customer-submitted reports of patient safety issues, some appointing a formal team to guide follow-on actions. However, when asked about the volume and types of adverse events related to their EHR products, vendor responses ranged from 0 to 40 events per year, although none provided a full list of problematic events and potential patient safety concerns (IOM, 2011). The committee considered all these statements over the course of its deliberations and weighed them against the literature and its expertise. Given the committee's limited ability to verify statements from the public and vendors, it did not systematically weigh these statements.

RECOMMENDATIONS FROM PREVIOUS IOM REPORTS REGARDING HEALTH IT

For more than two decades, the IOM and the National Academy of Sciences have recognized health IT as a central component of a safe, high-quality health care system. The first uses of computers for medical information and records were primarily for reporting the results of laboratory tests and for administrative purposes, particularly billing. It was only later that they began to be used for a wider array of clinical uses, in particular as a supplement to or replacement for paper for holding medical record data. The growth of computing technology led the IOM to form a committee in

---

[4] In this report, the term vendor is used to mean companies that design, make, and sell health IT products. In many industries the terms developers and manufacturers are also used, but in health IT, vendor is generally the preferred term.

1989 to examine this development and make recommendations relating to the future of computers in record keeping. The report of this committee was entitled *The Computer-Based Patient Record: An Essential Technology for Health Care* and it explained the contrast to the traditional paper-based medical record. Lawrence Weed had described his problem-oriented medical record in 1969 and it was being developed in a computer-based format in a system known as the problem-oriented medical information system (PROMIS). The IOM report made a number of important conceptual contributions well ahead of the maturation of the technology and its uses in health care by focusing first on the patient, making it clear that patient-centeredness was primary, and that the key was not who was entering the information into the record. Clearly, it denoted that the record was based upon a computer and not on paper. The subtitle focused upon *health care*, not medical, nursing, public health, or any other subcategory relating to health-related activities for which a record was kept. In that sense, it was not envisioning an *electronic medical record*, but a record for medical care as well as any care relating to health at that time.

Finally, *The Computer-Based Patient Record* identified a list of 12 functions that a record should properly serve. The committee's vision was very clear in the context of both its perspective and its functionalities. The report was also limited in the sense that computer-based personal health records and computer-based public health records have changed dramatically since the time of its publication. The report reflected its time with a focus upon the record as used in medical environments, but not solely for medicine or medical care in the narrowest sense. It set a vision for nationwide computer-based patient records and called for electronic records to be standard in care delivery and detailed primary and secondary uses of electronic records (IOM, 1991). A later effort concluded that development of robust data was critical to attaining this vision, requiring the creation of data standards and collection of data for regional and national patient-record efforts (IOM, 1994).

However, progress toward these goals was too slow (IOM, 2001), leading to the continued recognition that health IT is essential to reengineering the health care system (IOM, 2001, 2003, 2004b; NAE and IOM, 2005). Recommendations identified ways health IT could be advanced and included the following:

- A renewed call for comprehensive national data standards to be established and disseminated by the federal government for the definition, collection, coding, and exchange of data (IOM, 2001, 2004b);
- A series of demonstration projects to develop a health IT infrastructure—particularly in the areas of communication, access

to patient information, knowledge management, and decision support—that would take place at the community, state, multistate, and regional levels (IOM, 2003);

- Industry and government collaboration at a national level, for example with the development of public–private partnerships (IOM, 2004a; NAE and IOM, 2005); and
- Large federal investments to support the development of a national health information infrastructure to improve patient safety and health care delivery (IOM, 2002, 2004b; NAE and IOM, 2005).

In 2003, the IOM reported that emerging competencies for the future include knowledge, skills, and attitudes relating to (1) practice in teams, (2) use of evidence-based knowledge, (3) continuously improving quality, (4) patient-centered care, and (5) employing informatics. Education and training must go beyond simply educating current clinicians on how to use a specific EHR product. For safe delivery of health care in the future, health professionals need to know how to work in complex systems. Understanding health IT within the context of contemporary health reforms and challenges for improving safety and outcomes will be critical (IOM, 2004a).

Upon recognizing that many types of health IT exist to address many different purposes, and can vary by setting of care, the IOM examined specific components of health IT (IOM, 2004b). Particular emphasis was placed on EHRs and reduction of medication errors. To help move the field forward, the IOM described an EHR system as a system that "encompasses (1) longitudinal collection of electronic health information for and about persons, (2) electronic access to person- and population-level information by authorized users, (3) provision of knowledge and decision support systems, and (4) support for efficient processes for health care delivery" (IOM, 2004b). It identified eight key functionalities for EHR systems: health information and data, results management, order entry management, decision support, electronic communication and connectivity, patient support, administrative processes, and reporting and population health management.

In an effort to emphasize the importance of preventing medication errors, the effective use of technologies to reduce medication errors was the focus of a different IOM committee. Agencies within HHS were identified as actors to establish standards affecting drug-related health information technologies, such as development of a common drug nomenclature to be used in all clinical IT systems, specifications for alert mechanisms and intelligent prompting, and optimum design of user interfaces for the clinical environment. These recommendations were made to address patients' unique characteristics and needs while also recognizing providers' individual prescribing, ordering, and error patterns (IOM, 2006).

Despite the efforts made over the past few decades, a recent report by the National Research Council (NRC, 2009) concluded that the current investment in health IT is inadequate to fully realize the positive effects IT can have to make health care more effective. If the promise of a high-performing health care system is to be achieved, future efforts will need to emphasize cognitive support for health care providers and patients, such as enhanced decision making and problem solving, which will require an interdisciplinary approach. In essence, the report sought to refocus attention to humans and away from technology as a simple solution.

REPORT STRUCTURE

This report consists of seven chapters, of which this introduction is the first. The committee evaluates the current state of health IT in Chapter 2 and offers a systems approach for health IT safety in Chapter 3. Chapter 4 highlights opportunities to improve safety from the perspectives of both manufacturers and users of health IT. The role of patients and their families is explored in Chapter 5. The responsibilities of the private and public sectors are explored in Chapter 6. Finally, the committee offers a future research agenda for health IT safety in Chapter 7.

REFERENCES

AHRQ (Agency for Healthcare Research and Quality). 2009. *Electronic health record usability: Evaluation and use case framework*. Rockville, MD: AHRQ.

AHRQ. 2010. *National healthcare quality report*. Rockville, MD: AHRQ.

Aleccia, J. 2011. Nurse's suicide highlights twin tragedies of medical errors. MSNBC.com. http://www.msnbc.msn.com/id/43529641/ns/health-health_care/t/nurses-suicide-highlights-twin-tragedies-medical-errors/#.Tph_EHI2Y9Y (accessed October 14, 2011).

Associated Press. 2009. Veterans given wrong drug doses due to glitch. MSNBC.com. http://www.msnbc.msn.com/id/28655104/#.Tph-b3I2Y9Z (accessed October 14, 2011).

Bishop, T. F., A. K. Ryan, and L. P. Casalino. 2011. Paid malpractice claims for adverse events in inpatient and outpatient settings. *Journal of the American Medical Association* 305(23):2427-2431.

Blumenthal, D. 2010. Statement to IOM Committee on Patient Safety and Health Information Technology. Statement read at the Workshop of the IOM Committee on Patient Safety and Health Information Technology, Washington, DC.

Chassin, M. R., J. M. Loeb, S. P. Schmaltz, and R. M. Wachter. 2010. Accountability measures—using measurement to promote quality improvement. *New England Journal of Medicine* 363(7):683-688.

Classen, D. C., R. Resar, F. Griffin, F. Federico, T. Frankel, N. Kimmel, J. C. Whittington, A. Frankel, A. Seger, and B. C. James. 2011. "Global trigger tool" shows that adverse events in hospitals may be ten times greater than previously measured. *Health Affairs* 30(4):581-589.

Gandhi, T. K., and T. H. Lee. 2010. Patient safety beyond the hospital. *New England Journal of Medicine* 363(11):1001-1003.

Graham, J., and C. Dizikes. 2011. Baby's death spotlights safety risks linked to computerized systems. *Los Angeles Times*. http://www.latimes.com/health/ct-met-technology-errors-20110627,0,2158183.story (accessed June 29, 2011).

Hammons, T., N. F. Piland, S. D. Small, M. J. Hatlie, H. R. Burstin. 2001. *An agenda for research in ambulatory patient safety: Conference synthesis*. Rockville, MD: Agency for Healthcare Research and Quality.

HHS (Department of Health and Human Services). 2010a. *Adverse events in hospitals: National incidence among Medicare beneficiaries*. Washington, DC: HHS.

HHS. 2010b. Letter to the National Coordinator for Health Information Technology providing recommendations on the topic of patient safety. Washington, DC: HHS.

HHS. 2011. *News release: Partnership for patients to improve care and lower costs for Americans*. Washington, DC: HHS.

HIMSS (Healthcare Information and Management Systems Society). 2009. *Defining and testing EMR usability: Principles and proposed methods of EMR usability evaluation and rating*. http://www.himss.org/content/files/HIMSS_DefiningandTestingEMRUsability.pdf (accessed April 25, 2011).

Hsiao, C.-J., E. Hing, T. C. Socey, and B. Cai. 2010. *Electronic medical record/electronic health record systems of office-based physicians: United States, 2009, and preliminary 2010 state estimates*. Atlanta, GA: CDC.

IOM (Institute of Medicine). 1991. *The computer-based patient record: An essential technology for health care*. Washington, DC: National Academy Press.

IOM. 1994. *Health data in the information age: Use, disclosure, and privacy*. Washington, DC: National Academy Press.

IOM. 1999. *To err is human: Building a safer health system*. Washington, DC: National Academy Press.

IOM. 2001. *Crossing the quality chasm: A new health system for the 21st century*. Washington, DC: National Academy Press.

IOM. 2002. *Leadership by example: Coordinating government roles in improving health care quality*. Washington, DC: The National Academies Press.

IOM. 2003. *Fostering rapid advances in health care: Learning from system demonstrations*. Washington, DC: The National Academies Press.

IOM. 2004a. *1st annual Crossing the Quality Chasm Summit: A focus on communities*. Washington, DC: The National Academies Press.

IOM. 2004b. *Patient safety: Achieving a new standard for care*. Washington, DC: The National Academies Press.

IOM. 2006. *Preventing medication errors: Quality Chasm Series*. Washington, DC: The National Academies Press.

IOM. 2011 (unpublished). *Vendor responses—summary*. Washington, DC: IOM.

Jha, A. K., C. M. DesRoches, P. D. Kralovec, and M. S. Joshi. 2010. A progress report on electronic health records in U.S. hospitals. *Health Affairs* 29(10):1951-1957.

Landrigan, C. P., G. J. Parry, C. B. Bones, A. D. Hackbarth, D. A. Goldmann, and P. J. Sharek. 2010. Temporal trends in rates of patient harm resulting from medical care. *New England Journal of Medicine* 363(22):2124-2134.

Lorincz, C. Y., E. Drazen, P. E. Sokol, K. V. Neerukonda, J. Metzger, M. C. Toepp, L. Maul, D. C. Classen, M. K. Wynia. 2011. *Research in ambulatory patient safety 2000–2010: A 10-year review*. Chicago, IL: American Medical Association.

McGlynn, E. A., S. M. Asch, J. Adams, J. Keesey, J. Hicks, A. DeCristofaro, and E. A. Kerr. 2003. The quality of health care delivered to adults in the United States. *New England Journal of Medicine* 348(26):2635-2645.

NAE (National Academy of Engineering) and IOM. 2005. *Building a better delivery system: A new engineering/health care parternship*. Washington, DC: The National Academies Press.

NCVHS (National Committee on Vital and Health Statistics). 2001. *Information for health: A strategy for building the National Health Information Infrastructure.* Washington, DC: NCVHS.

Neily, J., P. D. Mills, Y. Young-Xu, B. T. Carney, P. West, D. H. Berger, L. M. Mazzia, D. E. Paull, and J. P. Bagian. 2010. Association between implementation of a medical team training program and surgical mortality. *Journal of the American Medical Association* 304(15):1693-1700.

NRC (National Research Council). 2009. *Computational technology for effective health care: Immediate steps and strategic directions.* Washington, DC: The National Academies Press.

ONC (Office of the National Coordinator for Health IT). 2011. *Federal advisory committees (FACAs).* http://healthit.hhs.gov/portal/server.pt/community/healthit_hhs_gov__federal_advisory_committees_(facas)/1149#top (accessed February 4, 2011).

PCAST (President's Council of Advisors on Science and Technology). 2010. *Realizing the full potential of health information technology to improve healthcare for Americans: The path forward.* http://www.whitehouse.gov/sites/default/files/microsites/ostp/pcast-health-it-report.pdf (accessed May 18, 2011).

Schulte, F., and E. Schwartz. 2010. As doctors shift to electronic health systems, signs of harm emerge. Huffington Post Investigative Fund. http://huffpostfund.org/stories/2010/04/doctors-shift-electronic-health-systems-signs-harm-emerge (accessed October 13, 2010).

Silver, J. D., and S. D. Hamill. 20111. Doctor, nurse disciplined by UPMC in kidney transplant case. Post-Gazette.com. http://www.post-gazette.com/pg/11147/1149429-114-0.stm#ixzz1amZZEw6Y (accessed October 14, 2011).

U.S. News. 2011. E-prescribing doesn't slash errors, study finds. *U.S. News and World Report.* http://health.usnews.com/health-news/family-health/articles/2011/06/30/e-prescribing-doesnt-slash-errors--study-finds (accessed October 14, 2011).

Whalen, J. 2011. U.K. ends health-service IT upgrade. *Wall Street Journal.* http://online.wsj.com/article/SB20001424053111904563904576587054273647780.html (accessed October 12, 2011).

Woods, D., S. Dekker, R. Cook, L. Johannesen, and N. Sarter. 2010. *Behind human error,* 2nd ed. Burlington, VT: Ashgate Publishing.

2

Evaluating the Current State of Patient Safety and Health IT

Health IT creates new opportunities to improve patient safety that do not exist in paper-based systems. For example, paper-based systems cannot detect and alert clinicians of drug–drug interactions, whereas electronic clinical decision support systems can. As a result, the expectations for safer care may be higher in a health IT–enabled environment as compared to a paper-based environment. However, implementation of health IT products does not automatically improve patient safety. In fact, health IT can be a contributing factor to adverse events, such as the overdosing of patients because of poor user interface design, failing to detect life threatening illnesses because of unclear information displays, and delays in treatment because of the loss of data. Adverse events, such as these, have lead to serious injuries and death (Aleccia, 2011; Associated Press, 2009; Graham and Dizikes, 2011; Schulte and Schwartz, 2010; Silver and Hamill, 2011; U.S. News, 2011).

The way in which health IT is designed, implemented, and used can determine whether it is an effective tool for improving patient safety or a hindrance that threatens patient safety and causes patient harm (see Box 2-1). The implementation of health IT, particularly complex health IT products, may result in less efficient systems and not give clinicians the flexibility they need to deliver the safest care possible (Greenhalgh et al., 2008). Currently, the relationship between these unintended consequences and the design, implementation, and use are not well understood.

This chapter uses the literature and experiences of health professionals to evaluate the impact of health IT on patient safety. The first several sections of this chapter discuss the challenges faced by health IT researchers by

BOX 2-1
Unintended Consequences of Health IT:
A Look at Implementing CPOE

Two pediatric intensive care units (ICUs) implemented the same electronic health record (EHR) system with computerized provider order entry (CPOE) in Pittsburgh and Seattle. The Pittsburgh experience led to a significant increase in mortality, while the same system implemented in Seattle did not (Del Beccaro et al., 2006; Han et al., 2005). Later, several other children's hospitals introduced the same CPOE system, leading to no change or even lower rates in mortality (Longhurst et al., 2010).

The differing impact on mortality rates may be due to the hospitals' differences in the implementation and use of the CPOE system. These differences, as illustrated by the Pittsburgh and Seattle pediatric ICUs, are highlighted below:

Pittsburgh

- Specific order sets designed for critical care were not created.
- Changes in workflow were not sufficiently predicted, resulting in a breakdown of communication between nurses and physicians.
- Orders for patients arriving via critical care transportation could not be written before the patients arrived at the hospital, delaying lifesaving treatments.
- Changes, unrelated to the CPOE system, were made in the administration and dispensing of medication that further frustrated the clinical staff, for example:
  o At the same time the CPOE system was installed, the satellite pharmacy serving the neonatal ICU was closed and medications had to be obtained from the central pharmacy, delaying treatment.
  o Emergency prescriptions were required to be preapproved, and all drugs were moved to the central pharmacy.

Seattle

- Researchers visited Pittsburgh to learn about problems associated with their implementation of the CPOE system.
- Intensive care staff was actively involved during the design, build, and implementation stages.
- Specific order sets were designed for ICU and pediatric ICU before implementation.
- New order sets, based on the most frequently used orders, were created to help reduce the time it takes a clinician to enter orders (Del Beccaro et al., 2006; Han et al., 2005).

detailing the complexity of health IT and patient safety, the limitations in the literature to determine health IT's impact on patient safety, and how the magnitude of harm is masked. The chapter then analyzes the literature to determine how individual components of health IT have impacted patient safety and how data from health IT can be leveraged to improve safety in different populations. Next, it describes how policy makers can learn from health IT experiences from abroad.

COMPLEXITY OF HEALTH IT AND PATIENT SAFETY

In general, health IT is not a specific product but is composed of components—such as computerized provider order entry (CPOE) systems and clinical decision support (CDS) systems—that are designed, implemented, and used differently by various vendors, health care settings, and users (Hayrinen et al., 2008). These differences can have dramatic effects on care processes including care design, workflow, and—ultimately—the quality and safety of the care delivered. When health IT is designed and implemented in a manner that complements how information is transferred between health professionals and patients, the reliability of patient information—and therefore patient safety—can increase (Dorr et al., 2007; Niazkhani et al., 2009; Shah et al., 2006). However, when health IT unexpectedly alters workflow, it has the potential to hinder clinicians' abilities to communicate patient information (Niazkhani et al., 2009), and it may result in increased cognitive workload, clinicians ignoring computer-generated information, continued reliance on various traditional modes of communication, creation of unsafe workarounds, and more time spent dealing with health IT than with patient care (Ash et al., 2009). Several important factors regarding how health IT products are designed and implemented can have meaningful effects on the collection, storage, and transfer of information, as well as the utility of the product. Slight variations in these factors can have differing effects on how health IT impacts patient safety. Some of these factors include the following:

- Decisions about implementation strategies (e.g., "big bang" versus incremental);
- The degree to which users can configure their IT system and the approaches to such configurations;
- Clinician training strategies;
- Frontline use (e.g., the IT integration into and redesign of clinical workflow); and
- Tools for analyzing and reporting results of care (e.g., quality improvement).

LIMITATIONS OF CURRENT LITERATURE TO DETERMINE
HEALTH IT'S IMPACT ON PATIENT SAFETY

Like all studies regarding patient safety, studies focusing on health IT and patient safety are complex and subject to a variety of methodological challenges. To provide generalizable knowledge about the impact of health IT on patient safety, the interaction of the factors listed in the previous section (e.g., frontline use) needs to be understood. However, very few studies to date have done so, resulting in major gaps in our knowledge regarding how health IT affects safety. While most of the literature examining the effects of health IT has focused on quality and processes of care, studies regarding the impact of health IT on patient safety have been narrowly focused on a few specific aspects of care. Given that adverse events (events resulting in unintended harm to a patient from a medical intervention [IOM, 2004]) are multifaceted and diverse, much of the literature that does center on how health IT affects patient safety has focused on prevention of medication errors, identification of patients at high risk for adverse events, and avoidance of documentation errors. Although much of this evidence suggests that IT can be helpful in improving patient safety, a number of studies have failed to find a benefit (Black et al., 2011; Culler et al., 2006; Garg et al., 2005; Reckmann et al., 2009).

Many studies, including meta-analyses, offer strong evidence that computerization of prescribing can dramatically improve patient safety. These products were consistently correlated with lowering the frequency of medication errors and may be able to reduce preventable adverse drug events significantly (Kaushal et al., 2003; Shamliyan et al., 2008; Wolfstadt et al., 2008). However, the degree to which health IT can lower medication errors varies widely among the different computerized prescribing systems used (Nanji et al., 2011).

The evidence of similar impact outside of medication safety is much weaker (Bates and Gawande, 2003). Indeed, some systematic reviews conclude that the current literature is insufficient to establish any beneficial impact of health IT on patient safety and health outcomes (Black et al., 2011; Garg et al., 2005; Reckmann et al., 2009). More recently, new data have emerged, suggesting that health IT can introduce new patient safety challenges into the health care system (Magrabi et al., 2010, 2011). These studies are unable to accurately quantify the number of people harmed by health IT. This inability of the committee to quantify the harm makes it difficult to understand the tradeoffs between the potential safety benefits and harms caused by health IT.

The differing results found in the literature may be due to a variety of reasons. Among those reasons are the heterogeneous nature of health IT—including the differences in the products themselves, how they are implemented, and how they are used across care settings. Most studies focused on health IT and patient safety examined care at a single medical center, often with homegrown IT systems. Aggregating many single-center studies, such as those common throughout the literature, does not necessarily lead to the same outcomes as having a few studies that are conducted in a broader array of clinical settings. However, systematic reviews have attempted to aggregate these studies and have done so in inconsistent ways, often choosing to include low-quality studies while failing to include higher-quality ones. Therefore, the committee could not point to any systematic reviews or studies as representing the most definitive evidence of the impact of health IT on patient safety (see Table B-1).

A major challenge in quantifying the harm that might result from health IT is the lack of data in this area. However, the absence of quantifiable evidence of health IT's harm is not evidence that health IT does not create harm. It is clear that harm exists. The current literature does not sufficiently produce estimates on the harm that might result from health IT. For example, a recent study by Nanji et al. evaluated the frequency, types, and causes of errors associated with outpatient computer-generated prescriptions. The study evaluated 3,850 prescriptions and found 466 errors, involving almost 12 percent of the orders. Because the error rates varied widely between different computerized prescribing systems (from 5.1 to 37.5 percent), the authors strongly recommended that users evaluate the safety of each system (Nanji et al., 2011). However, the authors were not allowed to list which error rates and safety issues were associated with each particular system. Instead, the article prescribed a "vigorous vendor selection" process, which each potential user would have to go through in order to identify safety concerns of that system. Had the authors been allowed to identify specific systems with higher error rates, users could know which systems to avoid and could select systems with characteristics that would best fit their workflow and safety needs.

Studies with generic descriptions of health IT products and patient safety issues will be of little utility to users because health IT products—even those made by the same manufacturers—are heterogeneous, tailored to individual clinical settings, and have varying impacts on patient safety. Therefore, to assist users in selecting the safest health IT product for their unique clinical environment, studies need to be able to name specific health IT products, describe how those products have been implemented, and identify their impact on patient safety in different clinical environments. For example, as mentioned in Box 2-1, a Pittsburgh pediatric intensive care unit's (ICU's) implementation of a CPOE system resulted in higher mortality; however, several different hospitals were able to subsequently identify safety problems associated with Pittsburgh's experience and implemented the same CPOE system with either no change or up to a 20 percent decrease in hospital-wide patient mortality (Longhurst et al., 2010). In order to identify problems associated with the Pittsburgh implementation, a pediatric ICU in Seattle sent researchers to Pittsburgh's facilities, met with their administrative and clinical leadership, and spoke with clinical staff. After months of correspondence, the Seattle pediatric ICU was able to determine why Pittsburgh's implementation resulted in a higher mortality rate and was able to avoid such problems (Del Beccaro et al., 2006; Han et al., 2005). When selecting health IT products, many potential users do not have the time or the resources to spend months corresponding, visiting, and observing other hospitals. Users and researchers need to be encouraged to provide specific descriptions of safety problems associated with particular health IT products in order to provide potential users with credible data regarding which IT products are safer than others.

BARRIERS TO KNOWING THE MAGNITUDE OF THE HARM

When researchers, consumer groups, and users attempt to identify and share information on health IT features related to adverse events and patient safety risks, they can be faced with barriers created by market inefficiencies within health IT, such as lack of information available to consumers and the inability of users to freely move between health IT products. For example, because the impact of health IT in each clinical environment is extremely diverse and highly dependent on the user's specific clinical environment, it is difficult for clinicians to know how the myriad of different health IT products will affect patient safety. Additionally, because of the substantial costs and effort used in tailoring and integrating health IT products, users may not be able to readily switch products after discovering patient safety problems. Many health IT products can only be maintained by the manufacturer of that product, causing users to maintain service contracts with that manufacturer, regardless of whether that manufacturer addresses patient safety issues associated with its product. Even if users are willing to switch health IT products, there is no guarantee another product will achieve greater levels of patient safety, once integrated. These inefficiencies result in an inadequate understanding of how health IT impacts patient safety and leads users to select and make a long-term commitment to products that may not adequately complement their clinical environment.

To increase understanding of how health IT affects patient safety and allows users to make informed decisions, it is important that the health IT community share details, such as screenshots of risk-enhancing interfaces, descriptions of potentially unsafe processes, and other components of health IT products associated with adverse events. Some vendors allow users to share information through industry conferences, sponsored user group meetings, blogs, and consultants that provide conduits for information about vendor experiences. However, the ability of users and researchers to share such information outside industry-controlled venues can be limited by nondisclosure clauses.

Nondisclosure clauses—commonly found in many types of commercial contracts and almost always included in software license agreements—are intended to protect licensors' intellectual property interests, competitive edge, and liability from consumer misuse of their products[1] (Koppel and Kreda, 2009). The fear of violating nondisclosure clauses and intellectual property interests may discourage users from sharing health IT–related patient safety risks. Additionally, if users believe that hold-harmless clauses, which are placed in many vendor contracts, can shift the liability of unsafe health IT features solely to the user, they may fear that disclosing unsafe features may unfairly increase their risk of liability.

To adequately understand how health IT impacts patient safety, users and researchers need to be able to share information that may normally be protected by intellectual property rights or may expose users to unfair liability. Some vendors have expended considerable effort to ensure patient safety, but allowing the disclosure of patient safety issues may cause vendors to lose their competitive advantage. Thus, some vendors may impose or enforce such restrictions in ways that may conceal patient safety issues[2] (Koppel and Kreda, 2009). As long as vendors may restrict the release of information about safety issues through confidentiality clauses, intellectual property protections, and hold-harmless clauses, the health care community will be limited in its understanding of how health IT affects patient safety.

Because the nature of these legal issues limits publicly available information, very little evidence establishes their frequency of use or impact on users (Koppel and Kreda, 2009). However, the committee believes that these types of contractual restrictions limit transparency, which significantly contributes to the gaps in knowledge of health IT–related patient safety risks. Regardless of whether these barriers have actually been used to prevent reporting, the fear of legal action itself may prevent health professionals from sharing crucial health IT–related information with researchers, consumer groups, other users, and the government. As stated by the American Medical Informatics Association, such clauses should be considered unethical (Goodman et al., 2011).

---

[1] Personal communication, B. Leshine, LeClairRyan, April 20, 2011; personal communication, H. Levine, Blaszak, Block & Boothby, LLP, June 10, 2011.

[2] Personal communication, B. Leshine, LeClairRyan, April 20, 2011; personal communication, H. Levine, Blaszak, Block & Boothby, LLP, June 10, 2011.

IMPACT OF HEALTH IT COMPONENTS ON PATIENT SAFETY

The following sections examine how individual components of health IT affect patient safety. However, most health IT products are not a single component, but a complex system of health IT components, sometimes collectively referred to as electronic health records (EHRs). Although the definition of EHRs can vary substantially, there are generally four core components of an EHR: electronic clinical documentation (usually physician, nurse, and other clinician documentation), electronic prescribing (e.g., computerized provider order entry), results reporting and management (e.g., clinical data repository), and clinical decision support (DesRoches et al., 2008; Jha et al., 2006, 2009a, 2009b). Many EHRs also include barcoding systems and patient engagement tools. The Office of the National Coordinator for Health Information Technology (ONC) defines an EHR as "a real-time patient health record with access to evidence-based decision support tools that can be used to aid clinicians in decision-making. The EHR can automate and streamline a clinician's workflow, ensuring that all clinical information is communicated. It can also prevent delays in response that result in gaps in care. The EHR can also support the collection of data for uses other than clinical care, such as billing, quality management, outcome reporting, and public health disease surveillance and reporting" (HHS, 2004; ONC, 2009).

Although EHR and health IT are terms that are still evolving and are often interpreted differently, much of the evidence regarding the impact of EHRs on patient safety has focused on individual components of EHRs. The following sections explore the evidence for individual components and then discuss the evidence from studies that use the "EHR" as a general term.[3] Because almost every component uses documentation and results review and management throughout their tasks (bar-coding, CPOE, and CDS systems all use documentation and results reporting and management in prescribing and delivering medication), this chapter will not address documentation results reporting and management individually. The section then looks at how current EHR systems can be leveraged to further improve patient safety. Table 2-1 summarizes the benefits and safety concerns commonly found in the literature.

---

[3] Although there are many other components of health IT, the bulk of the literature has focused on the following components: EHR, CPOE systems, CDS systems, patient engagement tools, and bar-coding systems. Some other components not listed in this chapter include medication reconciliation systems and smartpumps; see Appendix B.

TABLE 2-1
Potential Benefits and Safety Concerns of Health IT Components

Computerized Provider Order Entry (CPOE)

An electronic system that allows providers to record, store, retrieve, and modify orders (e.g., prescriptions, diagnostic testing, treatment, and/or radiology/imaging orders).

Potential Benefits	**Safety Concerns**

- Large increases in legible orders
- Shorter order turnaround times
- Lower relative risk of medication errors
- Higher percentage of patients who attain their treatment goals
	- Increases relative risk of medication errors
	- Increased ordering time
	- New opportunities for errors, such as:
	  • fragmented displays preventing a coherent view of patients' medications
	  • inflexible ordering formats generating wrong orders
	  • separations in functions that facilitate double dosing
	  • incompatible orders
	- Disruptions in workflow

Clinical Decision Support (CDS)

Monitors and alerts clinicians of patient conditions, prescriptions, and treatment to provide evidence-based clinical suggestions to health professionals at the point of care.

Potential Benefits	**Safety Concerns**

- Reductions in:
  • relative risk of medication errors
  • risk of toxic drug levels
  • time to therapeutic stabilization
  • management errors of resuscitating patients in adult trauma centers
  • prescriptions of nonpreferred medications
- Can effectively monitor and alert clinicians of adverse conditions
- Improve long-term treatment and increase the likelihood of achieving treatment goals
	- Rate of detecting drug–drug interactions varies widely among different vendors
	- Increases in mortality rate
	- High override rate of computer generated alerts (alert fatigue)

continued

TABLE 2-1 *Continued*

Bar-coding

Bar-coding can be used to track medications, orders, and other health care products. It can also be used to verify patient identification and dosage.

Potential Benefits

– Significant reductions in relative risk of medication errors associated with:
  • transcription
  • dispensing
  • administration errors

Safety Concerns

– Introduction of workarounds; for example, clinicians can:
  • scan medications and patient identification without visually checking to see if the medication, dosing, and patient identification are correct
  • attach patient identification bar-codes to another object instead of the patient
  • scan orders and medications of multiple patients at once instead of doing it each time the medication is dispensed

Patient Engagement Tools

Tools such as patient portals, smartphone applications, email, and interactive kiosks, which enable patients to participate in their health care treatment.

Potential Benefits

– Reduction in hospitalization rates in children

– Increases in patients' knowledge of treatment and illnesses

Safety Concerns

– Reliability of data entered by:
  • patients,
  • families,
  • friends, or
  • unauthorized users

NOTE: Table 2-1 is not intended to be an exhaustive list of all potential benefits and safety concerns associated with health IT. It represents the most common potential benefits and safety concerns.

Computerized Provider Order Entry

CPOE is an electronic system that allows providers to record, store, retrieve, and modify orders (e.g., prescriptions, diagnostic testing, treatment, and radiology/imaging orders). The use of CPOE has varying degrees of impact on patient safety, depending on how well the CPOE system complements or improves provider workflow. The successful impact of a CPOE system on patient safety may also depend heavily on the change management approach employed by organizational leadership to prepare clinicians and recipients of the new workflow, as well as the decision support tools associated with it. Short-term benefits of CPOE systems commonly found in studies include large increases in legible orders, shorter order turnaround times, lower relative risk of medication errors, and a higher percentage of patients who attain their treatment goals (Devine et al., 2010; Nam et al., 2007; Niazkhani et al., 2009). In the inpatient setting, a series of literature reviews and meta-analyses found that medication error rates fell (Kaushal et al., 2003; Shamliyan et al., 2008; Wolfstadt et al., 2008) due to the introduction of a CPOE system and most, though not all, studies suggest that the preventable adverse drug events (ADEs) rate decreases as well. Studies suggest that CPOE systems have a greater impact when designed for the specific needs of the hospital environment, workflow, and providers (Callen et al., 2010). For example, CPOE systems with order sets specifically designed for ICUs can increase efficiency and workflow (Ali et al., 2005).

Although the potential benefits of CPOE systems are well established, the harms that have been well articulated on a case-by-case basis have relatively little empirical basis behind them (Aleccia, 2011; Associated Press, 2009; Graham and Dizikes, 2011; Schulte and Schwartz, 2010; Silver and Hamill, 2011; U.S. News, 2011). The lack of data on harm is driven in large part, as described earlier, by practices that limit disclosure of health IT–related adverse drug events. Based on the existing information, it seems likely that, if these systems are either designed poorly or interface with clinicians in an ineffective manner, they can cause harm. Several experts have suggested that CPOE systems can have a number of potential adverse consequences, including increased ordering time, disruptions in workflow, new opportunities for errors (e.g., fragmented displays preventing a coherent view of patients' medications, inflexible ordering formats generating wrong orders, separations of functions that facilitate double dosing, and incompatible orders), and increased relative risk of medication errors (Koppel et al., 2005; Niazkhani et al., 2009; Santell et al., 2009; Singh et al., 2009; Walsh et al., 2006; Weant et al., 2007).

Some of the variability in the impact of CPOE systems is likely due to differences in decision support systems that can detect potential errors and/or generate care suggestions. For example, a CPOE system was introduced to a pediatric ICU without a CDS and resulted in no significant change in the rate of potential adverse drug events. However, a significant reduction in potential adverse drug events was found after a CDS system was implemented (Kadmon et al., 2009). Further discussion regarding the impact of CDS on patient safety is examined in the next section.

Clinical Decision Support

CDS systems are also an important component of an EHR. They can monitor patient conditions, prescriptions, and treatment to provide evidence-based clinical suggestions to health professionals at the point of care. The literature regarding the implementation of CDS is largely positive with respect to medication safety, though it is more mixed in domains such as chronic disease management. The majority of systematic reviews in this area report that most studies have demonstrated positive impacts on patient safety by improving practitioner performance and reducing the relative risk of medication errors, time to therapeutic stabilization, and risk of toxic drug levels (Ammenwerth et al., 2008; Conroy et al., 2007; Durieux et al., 2008; Garg et al., 2005; Georgiou et al., 2007). However, many of these reviews also stress that further research needs to be conducted to determine the full impact of CDS use on patient safety because many of the studies are often weak, differ substantially in their settings and design, and are inconsistent (Ammenwerth et al., 2008; Garg et al., 2005).

The inconsistency seen throughout the literature may be due to the differences in clinical settings, CPOE systems, CDS components, and workflow (Georgiou et al., 2007). Several studies have shown that the ability of CDS tools to perform even simple tasks, such as detecting drug–drug interactions, varies widely. For instance, when fictitious patients with simulated drug–drug interactions were entered in a CDS system, the results were disappointing. Using Leapfrog Group's "flight simulator technology," one study found that the mean scores for detecting simulated orders that would have led to serious adverse drug events for 62 hospitals was 43 percent (range 10 to 82 percent). The ability of the 62 hospitals to detect simulated medication errors that could result in fatalities was 53 percent (Metzger et al., 2010). In a similar study of 13 community and hospital pharmacies, six mock patients with a total of 37 drug–drug interactions were entered into each pharmacy's CDS e-prescribing system. The ability of the CDS systems to detect drug–drug interactions significantly varied. The CDS systems' sensitivity ranged from 0.15 to 0.94 and its specificity from 0.67 to 1.00, even among CDS systems designed by the same manufacturer (Abarca et al., 2006).

Although most of the literature suggests that CDS has had a positive overall impact on medication safety, a few studies have shown either no significant change with CDS use (Gandhi et al., 2005; Glassman et al., 2007; Gurwitz et al., 2005; Tierney et al., 2005) or negative consequences, such as increased patient mortality (see Box 2-1) (Han et al., 2005). However, these differences in impact may relate to variations in implementation and use of these systems, dissimilar designs, and how those CDS systems are used or differences in the organizations themselves (Del Beccaro et al., 2006). To create (or configure and populate) a CDS system to best improve patient safety, designers must consider hospitals' different clinical environments and test management practices (Callen et al., 2010). Several examples of successful implementations indicate that CDS systems may be more effective at increasing medication safety when they are specifically tailored to the clinical environment (Callen et al., 2010; Fitzgerald et al., 2011; Kadmon et al., 2009; Nies et al., 2010; Smith et al., 2006). For example, CDS use was found to be extremely effective at reducing management errors while resuscitating patients in an adult trauma center (Fitzgerald et al., 2011). Additionally, elderly patients were prescribed fewer nonpreferred medications after implementation of a CDS system specifically designed to alert and recommend clinicians of alternative treatments (Smith et al., 2006).

In addition to monitoring for potential medication errors, CDS systems can also suggest potential diagnoses and treatment, monitor patients' conditions, determine whether a potential or actual adverse event may occur, and alert clinicians to potential adverse conditions. Alerts can come in the form of chimes, flashing lights, and/or popup windows that appear while health professionals are accessing patient EHRs or entering orders into a computer system. Many alert systems require health professionals to acknowledge the alert by clicking a button in the popup window before continuing treatment, while others may appear and disappear without interrupting the health professionals' work. These systems can also help with surveillance and have been shown to be effective at diagnosing and alerting clinicians of adverse conditions (Claridge et al., 2009; Herasevich et al., 2009; Jha et al., 2008).

When implementing an alert system, success depends on how alerts impact workflow (Bates et al., 2003). If implemented correctly, alerts can improve patient safety. Alerts have been demonstrated to lower the rate of inappropriate medication prescriptions to select vulnerable populations, such as the elderly (Raebel et al., 2007). Flag alerts—reminders of patient diagnosis or conditions to clinicians who access patient EHRs—have been demonstrated to improve long-term treatment and increase the likelihood of achieving treatment goals (Agostini et al., 2007; Whitley et al., 2006). A retrospective analysis examining a diagnostic alarm system showed that the alarm system could detect and alert clinicians of critical events during anesthesia administration as effectively as anesthesiologists (Gohil et al., 2007).

Although patient safety can be improved by alerts, an improperly designed system may be ignored or even considered a nuisance to users (Phansalkar et al., 2010). In a retrospective cohort study of a large Veterans Affairs medical center and its five clinics, 10.2 percent of all alerts were unacknowledged and 6.8 percent of all alerts lacked timely follow-up (Singh et al., 2010). A controlled study of two medical departments in a French hospital showed that use of computer-generated alerts had no significant impact on the rate of inappropriate first prescriptions. Further analysis of the data showed that while the senior physicians made more inappropriate prescriptions with the alert system, residents made fewer inappropriate prescriptions, indicating that newer providers may be more adaptable to alert systems (Sellier et al., 2009).

Ineffectiveness of an alert system has been attributed to high rates of overrides and alert fatigue. If alerts are too numerous and are not representative of clinically significant conditions, they can overload clinical workflow and cause clinicians to ignore information that could prevent adverse events (Phansalkar et al., 2010). In an observational study, 25 percent of clinicians demonstrated signs of alert fatigue (van der Sijs et al., 2010). Several observational and retrospective studies found override rates between 80 and 98 percent (Lin et al., 2008; Shah et al., 2006; van der Sijs et al., 2009). Although high-severity alerts have a higher acceptance rate, they are still overridden more often than not (Isaac et al., 2009). One study was able to substantially reduce override rates of serious alerts by developing a tiered alert system, where alerts of less serious magnitude do not interrupt workflow. The more serious alerts caused a popup window to appear and forced the clinicians to acknowledge the alert (Shah et al., 2006). By limiting interruptions in workflow, an alert system can remind clinicians of important patient information without causing alert fatigue or high override rates.

Bar-Coding

The introduction of a bar-coding system to administer medication and verify patient identification has been strongly associated with significant reductions in relative risk of medication errors, including transcription, dispensing, and administration errors (Franklin et al., 2007; Poon et al., 2010). Although bar-coding has been shown to reduce medication errors, like any other technology, it can also create new opportunities for errors to occur. In a study observing and interviewing clinicians who use bar-coding systems to dispense and order medication, examples of multiple workarounds that could lead to patient harm were found. For example, clinicians who violate safe procedures and practices may scan medications and patient identification without visually checking to see if the medication, dosing, and patient are correct. Instead, clinicians depend on alarms or alerts to detect errors that may never have occurred if visually checked. An example of a workaround is that clinicians could attach patient identification bar-codes to another object instead of the patient, such as the patient's bed, which may lead to patients receiving incorrect medications in cases where the technology was perceived to be an obstacle to providing care. The study also found that, instead of scanning an order and the medication and then dispensing the medication to the patient, clinicians sometimes scanned all the orders and medications of multiple patients at once. This would save clinicians time because they would not have to scan the orders and medications each time they administered the medications. However, this workaround could result in the clinician giving patients wrong medications (Koppel et al., 2008). Despite the presence of these workarounds, the overall effect of bar-coding has been shown to substantially reduce the relative risk of medication errors, both at the point of care (Franklin et al., 2007; Poon et al., 2010) and in dispensing errors in the pharmacy (Poon et al., 2006).

Patient Engagement Tools

To date, much of the data on patient care reside on paper with little ability for patients and their families to access or use the information to improve their own health. Adoption of health IT by consumers is growing and includes a variety of tools that patients can use to engage in their care. These engagement tools are in varying stages of development and sophistication, with a growing number using smartphones as a common platform.

The literature regarding patient engagement tools generally does not focus on safety. Rather, the focus of most studies primarily examines the levels of comfort patients have with patient engagement tools and how engaged they are when these tools are made available to them. However, some studies demonstrate that patient engagement tools reduce hospitalization rates in children, increase patients knowledge of treatment and illnesses, and increase clinician knowledge (Murray et al., 2009; Ngo-Metzger et al., 2010).

Electronic Health Records

The following section discusses studies that focus either on EHRs as a whole or on how multiple components have affected patient safety. Implementation of EHRs has been reported to increase providers' perceptions of safety (Ferris et al., 2009), to lower infection rates (Parente and McCullough, 2009), and to reduce the number of documentation errors (Smith et al., 2009). While a review of the literature establishes that the use of EHRs improves process measures of quality of care in certain domains (e.g., preventions, specific chronic diseases), its impact on patient outcomes has been much more mixed (Einbinder and Bates, 2007).

The literature regarding EHR features, such as electronic documentation and results review and management, are also mixed. While health professionals perceive that these components can increase safety and efficiency (Ferris et al., 2009), they also expressed that features—such as copy and paste forward functions—can pose patient safety risks. One study found that the implementation of electronic vital sign documentation can reduce medical error rates in half (Gearing et al., 2006), while another study found that more than half of new aortic dilations discovered by computed tomography (CT) scan could not be found within patients' EHRs (Gordon et al., 2009).

The effectiveness of an EHR system on patient safety is dependent on the compatibility of that EHR with the individual needs of its users (Hayrinen et al., 2008). For example, EHR implementation can have differing effects on the flow of patient information (Benham-Hutchins and Effken, 2010). The Department of Veterans Affairs was able to demonstrate that an EHR could help coordinate care by providing a continuous flow of information among multiple clinicians (Litaker et al., 2005). Conversely, other studies in different clinical settings have found EHR implementation to have either no effect or a negative impact on workflow and patient outcomes (Benham-Hutchins and Effken, 2010; DesRoches et al., 2010). In a survey of an urban, university-based hospital, 84 percent of surveyed health professionals preferred verbal over electronic communication because they believed information contained in the EHR was unreliable. There, it was found that health professionals used nonlinear communication, combining several modes of communication to exchange patient information, including EHRs, paper notes, phone, and in-person verbal communication (Benham-Hutchins and Effken, 2010).

In general, EHRs have the potential to greatly increase patient safety, but the potential has not been realized consistently. For example, EHRs could include tools to help ensure that if a major issue such as an aortic aneurysm is detected, it is added to a problem list, or that problem and medication lists get updated more effectively. Research is needed to develop such tools, though early evidence suggests they have the potential to be highly effective (Wright et al., 2011). More broadly, additional research needs to be conducted on how various EHR designs affect different workflows and providers' needs.

LEVERAGING EHR DATA TO IMPROVE SAFETY OF POPULATIONS

In addition to results reporting for individual patients, EHRs can be a rich source of data for the identification of care gaps and patient lists for monitoring and clinical action across populations. While the degree of harm to patients is unclear, the failure to follow up on laboratory results represents one of the leading causes of lawsuits in the outpatient setting (Gandhi et al., 2006). Reports have shown that many abnormal lab results had not been acted upon by the appropriate clinicians, leading to important delays in diagnosis and treatment to patients (Kravitz et al., 1997; Magid et al., 2010). Surveys demonstrate that physicians are dissatisfied with paper approaches to management of test results (Poon et al., 2004). Data, identifying care gaps, and patient lists for monitoring, and clinical action across populations can be extracted from EHRs. Inpatient "system lists" of patients provide real-time data to monitor and identify high-risk patients for falls, pain management, pressure ulcers, ventilator-acquired pneumonia, and restraints. They can also be used to communicate test results directly to patients, which improves patient satisfaction (Matheny et al., 2007).

These population support tools have been shown to be effective at identifying gaps in care. Population support tools identified gaps in 32 evidence-based care recommendations for individual patients, groups of patients selected by a provider, or all patients on a primary care provider's panel. One tool was shown to have improved primary care teams' performance by up to 21 percent on preventive, monitoring, and therapeutic evidence-based recommendations (Zhou et al., 2011). A similar registry targeting females over the age 67 with a previous fracture along with follow-up activity showed a 13 to 44 percent improvement in patients receiving an evaluation and/or treatment for osteoporosis (Feldstein et al., 2007).

A powerful, more long-term impact was described in "The Best Medicine" (Begley, 2011). Begley describes the use of data from an EHR to find out which antihypertension drugs worked best if diuretics do not bring about the needed reduction in blood pressure (Begley, 2011). More proximate to patient safety is the early Kaiser Permanente recall of Vioxx. Here, Kaiser's EHR data independently showed increased incidence of heart attack and stroke. Based on these data, Kaiser stopped use of Vioxx months prior to the Merck recall (Graham et al., 2005).

Finally, EHRs can be used to detect, document, analyze, track, and report patient safety problems, including both adverse events and errors. Initially, automated EHRs were used to detect adverse drug events in hospital patients (Classen et al., 1991; Jha et al., 1998). This type of automated surveillance was expanded to health care–associated infections (Evans et al., 1998) and has been used increasingly by hospitals as the routine and operational approach to detecting these infections from ICU central line–related bloodstream infections to surgical-site infections that occur long after discharge (Wright, 2008). Recently, commercial EHRs that allow broad use of real-time safety tracking systems have been expanded to detect global adverse events in hospitalized patients (Classen et al., 2011). These EHR databases could also be retrospectively data-mined to study the occurrence of harm to patients across the continuum of care.

LESSONS FROM THE INTERNATIONAL COMMUNITY: INTERNATIONAL COMPARISONS

There are a significant number of high-income countries and multinational programs that have made substantial progress in implementing health IT and improving patient safety, at least in the ambulatory care setting. These countries can serve as important lessons from these settings for health professionals and policy makers in the United States. There has been a series of multinational programs to improve patient safety in which health IT has played a key role. For example, the World Health Organization's (WHO's) patient safety program has 13 specific patient safety action areas that focus on patient safety as a global health care issue. These action areas are aimed to "coordinate, disseminate, and accelerate improvements in patient safety worldwide" (WHO, 2011a). Although it focuses on a broad range of safety issues, "Action Area 8: Technology and Patient Safety," most specifically, targets systemic and technical aspects to improve patient safety around the world by promoting personal health records (PHRs), automated prescribing systems, simulation training, and failsafe mechanisms in diagnostic tools, such as computerized radiographs (WHO, 2008, 2011a, 2011b).

On a similarly large scale, the European Union (EU) has funded specific eHealth initiatives (EU, 2010a) and the use of technology to improve the quality and safety of care delivered during disaster response efforts (EU, 2007). These programs focus on PHRs, patient guidance services, virtual physiological humans, and computer simulations. The EU is supporting several efforts using information and communication technologies to improve patient safety, focusing on the "development of advanced applications to improve risk assessment and patient safety" (EU, 2010b). In 2009 alone, the EU invested €28 million (EU, 2010b), including programs such as Patient Safety through Intelligent Procedures in Medication (PSIP), whose main aim is to develop computer applications and to educate providers and patients on how to prevent medication errors (PSIP, 2011). Additionally, the Safety for Robotic Surgery (SAFROS) project seeks to develop technologies for patient safety in robotic surgery (SAFROS, 2009).

Broad country comparison studies have been conducted on the use of health IT and its potential to improve patient safety. For example, an international cross-sectional study examined health IT's functional capacity and quality of care delivered in Australia, Canada, Denmark, Germany, the Netherlands, New Zealand, the United Kingdom, and the United States. The study found that, when controlling for within country differences of specific health IT methods adopted and primary care physician (PCP) practice sizes, significant disparities exist in the quality of care delivered among practices with low IT capacity compared to those with high IT capacity. IT functional capacity was measured through a count of 14 different items (such as whether the clinician used an EHR, prescribed medicine electronically, and had a computerized system for patient reminders, prompts for potential drug interaction, and test results). Practices were deemed "low" if they had 2 or fewer of the 14 items and "high" if they had between 7 and 14 items (Davis et al., 2009).

Although the study focused on several outcomes, the specific safety outcome measured was whether a physician practice had a specific, documented process for patient follow-up and analysis of adverse events. Thirty-eight percent of physicians had a documented process for all adverse events (ranging from 27 percent of physicians in low-capacity countries to 43 percent in high-capacity countries), while 17 percent of physicians had a process for adverse drug reactions online (ranging from 22 percent in low-capacity countries to 15 percent in high-capacity countries) (Davis et al., 2009). Approximately 50 percent of practices with low IT capacity reported no processes for following up on adverse events compared to 41 percent of practices with higher IT functionality. Researchers suggested that countries that support a stronger IT infrastructure are better suited to address coordination of care and safety issues, as well as to maintain satisfaction among the PCP community (Davis et al., 2009).

Other country-specific studies have been conducted, including a series of papers comparing the adoption of health IT among PCP offices in New Zealand and Denmark, two countries leading the way in the adoption of health IT over the past two decades (Protti et al., 2008a, 2008b, 2008c, 2008d, 2009). These studies suggest that it has been possible for many nations to adopt and use health IT in PCP practices without measurable, deleterious consequences on patient safety.

Although the United States has made significant strides in health IT over the past 20 years, it is clear that many other high-income nations are much further ahead in IT adoption, at least in the ambulatory setting. Despite the fact that these other nations have had a much greater experience with health IT, there is very little direct information on the impact of their investments on patient safety. The primary lesson for the United States is that it is possible to have widespread adoption of health IT without harming safety. What the optimal strategies are for doing so cannot be so easily gleaned by looking at these other nations.

CONCLUSION

Health IT has already been shown to improve medication safety. Although the evidence is mixed for areas outside of medication safety, both within the United States and abroad, the fact that several studies have improved patient safety with implementation of health IT leads the committee to believe that health IT has at least the potential to drastically improve patient safety in other areas of care. As with any new technology, health IT carries benefits and risks of new and greater harms. To fully capitalize on the potential that health IT may have on patient safety, a more comprehensive understanding of how health IT impacts potential harms, workflow, and safety is needed.

REFERENCES

Abarca, J., L. R. Colon, V. S. Wang, D. C. Malone, J. E. Murphy, and E. P. Armstrong. 2006. Evaluation of the performance of drug-drug interaction screening software in community and hospital pharmacies. *Journal of Managed Care Pharmacy* 12(5):383-389.

Agostini, J. V., Y. Zhang, and S. K. Inouye. 2007. Use of a computer-based reminder to improve sedative-hypnotic prescribing in older hospitalized patients. *Journal of the American Geriatrics Society* 55(1):43-48.

Aleccia, J. 2011. Nurse's suicide highlights twin tragedies of medical errors. MSNBC.com. http://www.msnbc.msn.com/id/43529641/ns/health-health_care/t/nurses-suicide-highlights-twin-tragedies-medical-errors/#.Tph_EHI2Y9Y (accessed October 14, 2011).

Ali, N. A., H. S. Mekhjian, P. L. Kuehn, T. D. Bentley, R. Kumar, A. K. Ferketich, and S. P. Hoffmann. 2005. Specificity of computerized physician order entry has a significant effect on the efficiency of workflow for critically ill patients. *Critical Care Medicine* 33(1):110-114.

Ammenwerth, E., P. Schnell-Inderst, C. Machan, and U. Siebert. 2008. The effect of electronic prescribing on medication errors and adverse drug events: A systematic review. *Journal of the American Medical Informatics Association* 15(5):585-600.

Ash, J. S., D. F. Sittig, R. Dykstra, E. Campbell, and K. Guappone. 2009. The unintended consequences of computerized provider order entry: Findings from a mixed methods exploration. *International Journal of Medical Informatics* 78(Suppl 1):S69-S76.

Associated Press. 2009. Veterans given wrong drug doses due to glitch. MSNBC.com. http://www.msnbc.msn.com/id/28655104/#.Tph-b3I2Y9Z (accessed October 14, 2011).

Bates, D. W., and A. A. Gawande. 2003. Improving safety with information technology. *New England Journal of Medicine* 348(25):2526-2534.

Bates, D. W., G. J. Kuperman, S. Wang, T. Gandhi, A. Kittler, L. Volk, C. Spurr, R. Khorasani, M. Tanasijevic, and B. Middleton. 2003. Ten commandments for effective clinical decision support: Making the practice of evidence-based medicine a reality. *Journal of the American Medical Informatics Association* 10(6):523-530.

Begley, S. 2011. The best medicine: Cutting health costs with comparative effectiveness research. *Scientific American.* http://www.scientificamerican.com/article.cfm?id=the-best-medicine-july-11 (accessed August 5, 2011).

Benham-Hutchins, M. M., and J. A. Effken. 2010. Multi-professional patterns and methods of communication during patient handoffs. *International Journal of Medical Informatics* 79(4):252-267.

Black, A. D., J. Car, C. Pagliari, C. Anandan, K. Cresswell, T. Bokun, B. McKinstry, R. Procter, A. Majeed, and A. Sheikh. 2011. The impact of eHealth on the quality and safety of health care: A systematic overview. *Public Library of Science Medicine* 8(1).

Callen, J., R. Paoloni, A. Georgiou, M. Prgomet, and J. Westbrook. 2010. The rate of missed test results in an emergency department an evaluation using an electronic test order and results viewing system. *Methods of Information in Medicine* 49(1):37-43.

Claridge, J. A., J. F. Golob, A. M. A. Fadlalla, B. M. D'Amico, J. R. Peerless, C. J. Yowler, and M. A. Malangoni. 2009. Who is monitoring your infections: Shouldn't you be? *Surgical Infections* 10(1):59-64.

Classen, D. C., S. L. Pestotnik, R. S. Evans, and J. P. Burke. 1991. Computerized surveillance of adverse drug events in hospital patients. *Journal of the American Medical Association* 266(20):2847-2851.

Classen, D. C., R. Resar, F. Griffin, F. Federico, T. Frankel, N. Kimmel, J. C. Whittington, A. Frankel, A. Seger, and B. C. James. 2011. "Global trigger tool" shows that adverse events in hospitals may be ten times greater than previously measured. *Health Affairs* 30(4):581-589.

Conroy, S., D. Sweis, C. Planner, V. Yeung, J. Collier, L. Haines, and I. C. K. Wong. 2007. Interventions to reduce dosing errors in children—a systematic review of the literature. *Drug Safety* 30(12):1111-1125.

Culler, S. D., A. Atherly, S. Walczak, A. Davis, J. N. Hawley, K. J. Rask, V. Naylor, and K. E. Thorpe. 2006. Urban-rural differences in the availability of hospital information technology applications: A survey of Georgia hospitals. *Journal of Rural Health* 22(3):242-247.

Davis, K., M. M. Doty, K. Shea, and K. Stremikis. 2009. Health information technology and physician perceptions of quality of care and satisfaction. *Health Policy* 90(2-3):239-246.

Del Beccaro, M. A., H. E. Jeffries, M. A. Eisenberg, and E. D. Harry. 2006. Computerized provider order entry implementation: No association with increased mortality rates in an intensive care unit. *Pediatrics* 118(1):290-295.

DesRoches, C. M., E. G. Campbell, S. R. Rao, K. Donelan, T. G. Ferris, A. Jha, R. Kaushal, D. E. Levy, S. Rosenbaum, A. E. Shields, and D. Blumenthal. 2008. Electronic health records in ambulatory care—a national survey of physicians. *New England Journal of Medicine* 359(1):50-60.

DesRoches, C. M., E. G. Campbell, C. Vogeli, J. Zheng, S. R. Rao, A. E. Shields, K. Donelan, S. Rosenbaum, S. J. Bristol, and A. K. Jha. 2010. Electronic health records' limited successes suggest more targeted uses. *Health Affairs* 29(4):639-646.

Devine, E. B., R. N. Hansen, J. L. Wilson-Norton, N. M. Lawless, A. W. Fisk, D. K. Blough, D. P. Martin, and S. D. Sullivan. 2010. The impact of computerized provider order entry on medication errors in a multispecialty group practice. *Journal of the American Medical Informatics Association* 17(1):78-84.

Dorr, D., L. M. Bonner, A. N. Cohen, R. S. Shoai, R. Perrin, E. Chaney, and A. S. Young. 2007. Informatics systems to promote improved care for chronic illness: A literature review. *Journal of the American Medical Informatics Association* 14(2):156-163.

Durieux, P., L. Trinquart, I. Colombet, J. Niès, R. Walton, A. Rajeswaran, M. Rège-Walther, E. Harvey, and B. Burnand. 2008. Computerized advice on drug dosage to improve prescribing practice. *Cochrane Database of Systematic Reviews* (3):CD002894.

Einbinder, J. S., and D. W. Bates. 2007. Leveraging information technology to improve quality and safety. *Yearbook of Medical Informatics* 2007:22-29.

EU (European Union). 2007. *Managing disasters and emergencies.* http://ec.europa.eu/information_society/tl/qualif/safety/index_en.htm (accessed June 20, 2011).

EU. 2010a. *Research in eHealth.* http://ec.europa.eu/information_society/activities/health/research/index_en.htm (accessed June 20, 2011).

EU. 2010b. *Risk assessment and patient safety.* http://ec.europa.eu/information_society/activities/health/research/fp7ps/index_en.htm (accessed June 20, 2011).

Evans, R. S., S. L. Pestotnik, D. C. Classen, T. P. Clemmer, L. K. Weaver, J. F. Orme, J. F. Lloyd, and J. P. Burke. 1998. A computer-assisted management program for antibiotics and other antiinfective agents. *New England Journal of Medicine* 338(4):232-238.

Feldstein, A. C., W. M. Vollmer, D. H. Smith, A. Petrik, J. Schneider, H. Glauber, and M. Herson. 2007. An outreach program improved osteoporosis management after a fracture. *Journal of the American Geriatrics Society* 55(9):1464-1469.

Ferris, T. G., S. A. Johnson, J. P. T. Co, M. Backus, J. Perrin, D. W. Bates, and E. G. Poon. 2009. Electronic results management in pediatric ambulatory care: Qualitative assessment. *Pediatrics* 123(Suppl 2):S85-S91.

Fitzgerald, M., P. Cameron, C. Mackenzie, N. Farrow, P. Scicluna, R. Gocentas, A. Bystrzycki, G. Lee, G. O'Reilly, N. Andrianopoulos, L. Dziukas, D. J. Cooper, A. Silvers, A. Mori, A. Murray, S. Smith, Y. Xiao, D. Stub, F. T. McDermott, and J. V. Rosenfeld. 2011. Trauma resuscitation errors and computer-assisted decision support. *Archives of Surgery* 146(2):218-225.

Franklin, B. D., K. O'Grady, P. Donyai, A. Jacklin, and N. Barber. 2007. The impact of a closed-loop electronic prescribing and administration system on prescribing errors, administration errors and staff time: A before-and-after study. *Quality & Safety in Health Care* 16(4):279-284.

Gandhi, T. K., S. B. Bartel, L. N. Shulman, D. Verrier, E. Burdick, A. Cleary, J. M. Rothschild, L. L. Leape, and D. W. Bates. 2005. Medication safety in the ambulatory chemotherapy setting. *Cancer* 104(11):2477-2483.

Gandhi, T. K., A. Kachalia, E. J. Thomas, A. L. Puopolo, C. Yoon, T. A. Brennan, and D. M. Studdert. 2006. Missed and delayed diagnoses in the ambulatory setting: A study of closed malpractice claims. *Annals of Internal Medicine* 145(7):488-496.

Garg, A., N. Adhikari, H. McDonald, M. Rosas-Arellano, P. Devereaux, J. Beyene, J. Sam, and R. Haynes. 2005. Effects of computerized clinical decision support systems on practitioner performance and patient outcomes: A systematic review. *Journal of the American Medical Association* 293(10):1223-1238.

Gearing, P., C. M. Olney, K. Davis, D. Lozano, L. B. Smith, and B. Friedman. 2006. Enhancing patient safety through electronic medical record documentation of vital signs. *Journal of Healthcare Information Management* 20(4):40-45.

Georgiou, A., M. Williamson, J. I. Westbrook, and S. Ray. 2007. The impact of computerised physician order entry systems on pathology services: A systematic review. *International Journal of Medical Informatics* 76(7):514-529.

Glassman, P. A., P. Belperio, A. Lanto, B. Simon, R. Valuck, J. Sayers, and M. Lee. 2007. The utility of adding retrospective medication profiling to computerized provider order entry in an ambulatory care population. *Journal of the American Medical Informatics Association* 14(4):424-431.

Gohil, B., H. Gholamhosseini, M. J. Harrison, A. Lowe, and A. Al-Jumaily. 2007. *Intelligent monitoring of critical pathological events during anesthesia.* Paper presented at Annual International Conference of the IEEE Engineering in Medicine & Biology Society, Lyon, France.

Goodman, K. W., E. S. Berner, M. A. Dente, B. Kaplan, R. Koppel, D. Rucker, D. Z. Sands, P. Winkelstein, and the AMIA Board of Directors. 2011. Challenges in ethics, safety, best practices, and oversight regarding HIT vendors, their customers, and patients: A report of an AMIA special task force. *Journal of the American Medical Informatics Association* 18(1):77-81.

Gordon, J. R. S., T. Wahls, R. C. Carlos, I. I. Pipinos, G. E. Rosenthal, and P. Cram. 2009. Failure to recognize newly identified aortic dilations in a health care system with an advanced electronic medical record. *Annals of Internal Medicine* 151(1):21-27.

Graham, D. J., D. Campen, R. Hui, M. Spence, C. Cheetham, G. Levy, S. Shoor, and W. A. Ray. 2005. Risk of acute myocardial infarction and sudden cardiac death in patients treated with cyclo-oxygenase 2 selective and non-selective non-steroidal anti-inflammatory drugs: Nested case-control study. *The Lancet* 365(9458):475-481.

Graham, J., and C. Dizikes. 2011. Baby's death spotlights safety risks linked to computerized systems. *Los Angeles Times.* http://www.latimes.com/health/ct-met-technology-errors-20110627,0,2158183.story (accessed June 29, 2011).

Greenhalgh, T., K. Stramer, T. Bratan, E. Byrne, Y. Mohammad, and J. Russell. 2008. Introduction of shared electronic records: Multi-site case study using diffusion of innovation theory. *British Medical Journal* 337:a1786.

Gurwitz, J. H., T. S. Field, J. Judge, P. Rochon, L. R. Harrold, C. Cadoret, M. Lee, K. White, J. LaPrino, J. Erramuspe-Mainard, M. DeFlorio, L. Gavendo, J. Auger, and D. W. Bates. 2005. The incidence of adverse drug events in two large academic long-term care facilities. *American Journal of Medicine* 118(3):251-258.

Han, Y. Y., J. A. Carcillo, S. T. Venkataraman, R. S. B. Clark, R. S. Watson, T. C. Nguyen, H. Bayir, and R. A. Orr. 2005. Unexpected increased mortality after implementation of a commercially sold computerized physician order entry system. *Pediatrics* 116(6):1506-1512.

Hayrinen, K., K. Saranto, and P. Nykanen. 2008. Definition, structure, content, use and impacts of electronic health records: A review of the research literature. *International Journal of Medical Informatics* 77(5):291-304.

Herasevich, V., M. Yilmaz, H. Khan, R. D. Hubmayr, and O. Gajic. 2009. Validation of an electronic surveillance system for acute lung injury. *Intensive Care Medicine* 35(6):1018-1023.

HHS (U.S. Department of Health and Human Services). 2004. *Health IT strategic framework: Glossary of selected terms* (accessed May 9, 2011).

IOM (Institute of Medicine). 2004. *Patient safety: Achieving a new standard for care.* Washington, DC: The National Academies Press.

Isaac, T., J. S. Weissman, R. B. Davis, M. Massagli, A. Cyrulik, D. Z. Sands, and S. N. Weingart. 2009. Overrides of medication alerts in ambulatory care. *Archives of Internal Medicine* 169(3):305-311.

Jha, A. K., G. J. Kuperman, J. M. Teich, L. Leape, B. Shea, E. Rittenberg, E. Burdick, D. L. Seger, M. V. Vliet, and D. W. Bates. 1998. Identifying adverse drug events. *Journal of the American Medical Informatics Association* 5(3):305-314.

Jha, A. K., T. G. Ferris, K. Donelan, C. DesRoches, A. Shields, S. Rosenbaum, and D. Blumenthal. 2006. How common are electronic health records in the United States? A summary of the evidence. *Health Affairs* 25(6):w496-w507.

Jha, A. K., J. Laguette, A. Seger, and D. W. Bates. 2008. Can surveillance system identify and avert adverse drug events? A prospective evaluation of a commercial application. *Journal of the American Medical Informatics Association* 15(5):647-653.

Jha, A. K., C. M. DesRoches, E. G. Campbell, K. Donelan, S. R. Rao, T. G. Ferris, A. Shields, S. Rosenbaum, and D. Blumenthal. 2009a. Use of electronic health records in U.S. hospitals. *New England Journal of Medicine* 360(16):1628-1638.

Jha, A. K., E. J. Orav, and A. M. Epstein. 2009b. Preventing readmissions with improved hospital discharge planning. *New England Journal of Medicine* 361(27):2637-2645.

Kadmon, G., E. Bron-Harlev, E. Nahum, O. Schiller, G. Haski, and T. Shonfeld. 2009. Computerized order entry with limited decision support to prevent prescription errors in a PICU. *Pediatrics* 124(3):935-940.

Kaushal, R., K. G. Shojania, and D. W. Bates. 2003. Effects of computerized physician order entry and clinical decision support systems on medication safety: A systematic review. *Archives of Internal Medicine* 163(12):1409-1416.

Koppel, R., and D. Kreda. 2009. Health care information technology vendors' "hold harmless" clause. *Journal of the American Medical Association* 301(12):1276-1278.

Koppel, R., J. P. Metlay, A. Cohen, B. Abaluck, A. R. Localio, S. E. Kimmel, and B. L. Strom. 2005. Role of computerized physician order entry systems in facilitating medication errors. *Journal of the American Medical Association* 293(10):1197-1203.

Koppel, R., T. Wetterneck, J. L. Telles, and B. T. Karsh. 2008. Workarounds to barcode medication administration systems: Their occurrences, causes, and threats to patient safety. *Journal of the American Medical Informatics Association* 15(4):408-423.

Kravitz, R. L., J. E. Rolph, and L. Petersen. 1997. Omission-related malpractice claims and the limits of defensive medicine. *Medical Care Research and Review* 54(4):456-471.

Lin, C. P., T. H. Payne, W. P. Nichol, P. J. Hoey, C. L. Andreson, and J. H. Gennari. 2008. Evaluating clinical decision support systems: Monitoring CPOE order check override rates in the Department of Veterans Affairs' computerized patient record system. *Journal of the American Medical Informatics Association* 15(5):620-626.

Litaker, D., C. Ritter, S. Ober, and D. Aron. 2005. Continuity of care and cardiovascular risk factor management: Does care by a single clinician add to informational continuity provided by electronic medical records? *American Journal of Managed Care* 11(11):689-696.

Longhurst, C. A., L. Parast, C. I. Sandborg, E. Widen, J. Sullivan, J. S. Hahn, C. G. Dawes, and P. J. Sharek. 2010. Decrease in hospital-wide mortality rate after implementation of a commercially sold computerized physician order entry system. *Pediatrics* 126(1):14-21.

Magid, D. J., S. M. Shetterly, K. L. Margolis, H. M. Tavel, P. J. O'Connor, J. V. Selby, and P. M. Ho. 2010. Comparative effectiveness of angiotensin-converting enzyme inhibitors versus β-blockers as second-line therapy for hypertension. *Circulation: Cardiovascular Quality and Outcomes* 3(5):453-458.

Magrabi, F., S. Y. W. Li, R. O. Day, and E. Coiera. 2010. Errors and electronic prescribing: A controlled laboratory study to examine task complexity and interruption effects. *Journal of the American Medical Informatics Association* 17(5):575-583.

Magrabi, F., M.-S. Ong, W. Runciman, and E. Coiera. 2011. Using FDA reports to inform a classification for health information technology safety problems. *Journal of the American Medical Informatics Association* 19(1):45-53.

Matheny, M. E., T. K. Gandhi, E. J. Orav, Z. Ladak-Merchant, D. W. Bates, G. J. Kuperman, and E. G. Poon. 2007. Impact of an automated test results management system on patients' satisfaction about test result communication. *Archives of Internal Medicine* 167(20):2233-2239.

Metzger, J., E. Welebob, D. W. Bates, S. Lipsitz, and D. C. Classen. 2010. Mixed results in the safety performance of computerized physician order entry. *Health Affairs* 29(4):655-663.

Murray, E., J. Burns, T. S. See, R. Lai, and I. Nazareth. 2009. Interactive health communication applications for people with chronic disease. *Cochrane Database of Systematic Reviews* (1):CD004274.

Nam, H. S., S. W. Han, S. H. Ahn, J. Y. Lee, H. Y. Choi, I. C. Park, and J. H. Heo. 2007. Improved time intervals by implementation of computerized physician order entry-based stroke team approach. *Cerebrovascular Diseases* 23(4):289-293.

Nanji, K. C., J. M. Rothschild, C. Salzberg, C. A. Keohane, K. Zigmont, J. Devita, T. K. Gandhi, A. K. Dalal, D. W. Bates, and E. G. Poon. 2011. Errors associated with outpatient computerized prescribing systems. *Journal of the American Medical Informatics Association* 18(6):767-773.

Ngo-Metzger, Q., G. R. Hayes, Y. N. Chen, R. Cygan, and C. F. Garfield. 2010. Improving communication between patients and providers using health information technology and other quality improvement strategies: Focus on low-income children. *Medical Care Research and Review* 67(5):246S-267S.

Niazkhani, Z., H. Pirnejad, M. Berg, and J. Aarts. 2009. The impact of computerized provider order entry systems on inpatient clinical workflow: A literature review. *Journal of the American Medical Informatics Association* 16(4):539-549.

Nies, J., I. Colombet, E. Zapletal, F. Gillaizeau, P. Chevalier, and P. Durieux. 2010. Effects of automated alerts on unnecessarily repeated serology tests in a cardiovascular surgery department: A time series analysis. *Health Services Research* 10(1):70.

ONC (Office of the National Coordinator for Health Information Technology). 2009. *Health IT terms: Glossary of selected terms related to Health IT*. http://healthit.hhs.gov/portal/server.pt?open=512&mode=2&cached=true&objID=1256&PageID=15726 (accessed March 20, 2011).

Parente, S. T., and J. S. McCullough. 2009. Health information technology and patient safety: Evidence from panel data. *Health Affairs* 28(2):357-360.

Phansalkar, S., J. Edworthy, E. Hellier, D. L. Seger, A. Schedlbauer, A. J. Avery, and D. W. Bates. 2010. A review of human factors principles for the design and implementation of medication safety alerts in clinical information systems. *Journal of the American Medical Informatics Association* 17(5):493-501.

Poon, E. G., T. K. Gandhi, T. D. Sequist, H. J. Murff, A. S. Karson, and D. W. Bates. 2004. "I wish I had seen this test result earlier!": Dissatisfaction with test result management systems in primary care. *Archives of Internal Medicine* 164(20):2223-2228.

Poon, E. G., J. L. Cina, W. Churchill, N. Patel, E. Featherstone, J. M. Rothschild, C. A. Keohane, A. D. Whittemore, D. W. Bates, and T. K. Gandhi. 2006. Medication dispensing errors and potential adverse drug events before and after implementing bar code technology in the pharmacy. *Annals of Internal Medicine* 145(6):426-434.

Poon, E. G., C. A. Keohane, C. S. Yoon, M. Ditmore, A. Bane, O. Levtzion-Korach, T. Moniz, J. M. Rothschild, A. B. Kachalia, J. Hayes, W. W. Churchill, S. Lipsitz, A. D. Whittemore, D. W. Bates, and T. K. Gandhi. 2010. Effect of bar-code technology on the safety of medication administration. *New England Journal of Medicine* 362(18):1698-1707.

Protti, D., T. Bowden, and I. Johansen. 2008a. Adoption of information technology in primary care physician offices in New Zealand and Denmark, part 1: Healthcare system comparisons. *Informatics in Primary Care* 16:183-187.

Protti, D., T. Bowden, and I. Johansen. 2008b. Adoption of information technology in primary care physician offices in New Zealand and Denmark, part 2: Historical comparisons. *Informatics in Primary Care* 16:189-193.

Protti, D., T. Bowden, and I. Johansen. 2008c. Adoption of information technology in primary care physician offices in New Zealand and Denmark, part 3: Medical record environment comparisons. *Informatics in Primary Care* 16:285-290.

Protti, D., T. Bowden, and I. Johansen. 2008d. Adoption of information technology in primary care physician offices in New Zealand and Denmark, part 4: Benefits comparisons. *Informatics in Primary Care* 16:291-296.

Protti, D., T. Bowden, and I. Johansen. 2009. Adoption of information technology in primary care physician offices in New Zealand and Denmark, part 5: Final comparisons. *Informatics in Primary Care* 17:17-22.

PSIP (Patient Safety through Intelligent Procedures in Medication). 2011. *PSIP: Patient safety through intelligent procedures in medication.* http://ec.europa.eu/information_society/activities/health/docs/projects/fp7/psip-factsheet.pdf (accessed June 25, 2011).

Raebel, M. A., J. Charles, J. Dugan, N. M. Carroll, E. J. Korner, D. W. Brand, and D. J. Magid. 2007. Randomized trial to improve prescribing safety in ambulatory elderly patients. *Journal of the American Geriatrics Society* 55(7):977-985.

Reckmann, M. H., J. I. Westbrook, Y. Koh, C. Lo, and R. O. Day. 2009. Does computerized provider order entry reduce prescribing errors for hospital inpatients? A systematic review. *Journal of the American Medical Informatics Association* 16(5):613-623.

SAFROS (Safety for Robotic Surgery). 2009. *The SAFROS project.* http://www.safros.eu/ (accessed June 27, 2011).

Santell, J. P., J. G. Kowiatek, R. J. Weber, R. W. Hicks, and C. A. Sirio. 2009. Medication errors resulting from computer entry by nonprescribers. *American Journal of Health-System Pharmacy* 66(9):843-853.

Schulte, F., and E. Schwartz. 2010. As doctors shift to electronic health systems, signs of harm emerge. Huffington Post Investigative Fund. http://huffpostfund.org/stories/2010/04/doctors-shift-electronic-health-systems-signs-harm-emerge (accessed October 13, 2010).

Sellier, E., I. Colombet, B. Sabatier, G. Breton, J. Nies, E. Zapletal, J. B. Arlet, D. Somme, and P. Durieux. 2009. Effect of alerts for drug dosage adjustment in inpatients with renal insufficiency. *Journal of the American Medical Informatics Association* 16(2):203-210.

Shah, N. R., A. C. Seger, D. L. Seger, J. M. Fiskio, G. J. Kuperman, B. Blumenfeld, E. G. Recklet, D. W. Bates, and T. K. Gandhi. 2006. Improving acceptance of computerized prescribing alerts in ambulatory care. *Journal of the American Medical Informatics Association* 13(1):5-11.

Shamliyan, T. A., S. Duval, J. Du, and R. L. Kane. 2008. Just what the doctor ordered. Review of the evidence of the impact of computerized physician order entry system on medication errors. *Health Services Research* 43(1 Pt 1):32-53.

Silver, J. D., and S. D. Hamill. 20111. Doctor, nurse disciplined by UPMC in kidney transplant case. Post-Gazette.com. http://www.post-gazette.com/pg/11147/1149429-114-0.stm#ixzz1amZZEw6Y (accessed October 14, 2011).

Singh, H., S. Mani, D. Espadas, N. Petersen, V. Franklin, and L. A. Petersen. 2009. Prescription errors and outcomes related to inconsistent information transmitted through computerized order entry: A prospective study. *Archives of Internal Medicine* 169(10):982-989.

Singh, H., E. J. Thomas, D. F. Sittig, L. Wilson, D. Espadas, M. M. Khan, and L. A. Petersen. 2010. Notification of abnormal lab test results in an electronic medical record: Do any safety concerns remain? *American Journal of Medicine* 123(3):238-244.

Smith, D. H., N. Perrin, A. Feldstein, X. H. Yang, D. Kuang, S. R. Simon, D. F. Sittig, R. Platt, and S. B. Soumerai. 2006. The impact of prescribing safety alerts for elderly persons in an electronic medical record—an interrupted time series evaluation. *Archives of Internal Medicine* 166(10):1098-1104.

Smith, L. B., L. Banner, D. Lozano, C. M. Olney, and B. Friedman. 2009. Connected care: Reducing errors through automated vital signs data upload. *Computers, Informatics, Nursing* 27(5):318-323.

Tierney, W. M., J. M. Overhage, M. D. Murray, L. E. Harris, X.-H. Zhou, G. J. Eckert, F. E. Smith, N. Nienaber, C. J. McDonald, and F. D. Wolinsky. 2005. Can computer-generated evidence-based care suggestions enhance evidence-based management of asthma and chronic obstructive pulmonary disease? A randomized, controlled trial. *Health Services Research* 40(2):477-497.

U.S. News. 2011. E-prescribing doesn't slash errors, study finds. *U.S. News and World Report.* http://health.usnews.com/health-news/family-health/articles/2011/06/30/e-prescribing-doesnt-slash-errors--study-finds (accessed October 14, 2011).

van der Sijs, H., A. Mulder, T. van Gelder, J. Aarts, M. Berg, and A. Vulto. 2009. Drug safety alert generation and overriding in a large Dutch university medical centre. *Pharmacoepidemiology and Drug Safety* 18(10):941-947.

van der Sijs, H., T. van Gelder, A. Vulto, M. Berg, and J. Aarts. 2010. Understanding handling of drug safety alerts: A simulation study. *International Journal of Medical Informatics* 79(5):361-369.

Walsh, K. E., W. G. Adams, H. Bauchner, R. J. Vinci, J. B. Chessare, M. R. Cooper, P. M. Hebert, E. G. Schainker, and C. P. Landrigan. 2006. Medication errors related to computerized order entry for children. *Pediatrics* 118(5):1872-1879.

Weant, K. A., A. M. Cook, and J. A. Armitstead. 2007. Medication-error reporting and pharmacy resident experience during implementation of computerized prescriber order entry. *American Journal of Health-System Pharmacy* 64(5):526-530.

Whitley, H. P., J. D. Fermo, and E. C. G. Chumney. 2006. 5-year evaluation of electronic medical record flag alerts for patients warranting secondary prevention of coronary heart disease. *Pharmacotherapy* 26(5):682-688.

WHO (World Health Organization). 2008. *World alliance for patient safety: Forward programme 2008-2009.* http://www.who.int/patientsafety/information_centre/reports/Alliance_Forward_Programme_2008.pdf (accessed June 27, 2011).

WHO. 2011a. *Patient safety: About us.* http://www.who.int/patientsafety/about/en/index.html (accessed June 25, 2011).

WHO. 2011b. *WHO patient safety—programme areas.* http://www.who.int/patientsafety/about/programmes/en/index.html (accessed June 25, 2011).

Wolfstadt, J. I., J. H. Gurwitz, T. S. Field, M. Lee, S. Kalkar, W. Wu, and P. A. Rochon. 2008. The effect of computerized physician order entry with clinical decision support on the rates of adverse drug events: A systematic review. *Journal of General Internal Medicine* 23(4):451-458.

Wright, A., J. Pang, J. C. Feblowitz, F. L. Maloney, A. R. Wilcox, H. Z. Ramelson, L. I. Schneider, and D. W. Bates. 2011. A method and knowledge base for automated inference of patient problems from structured data in an electronic medical record. *Journal of the American Medical Informatics Association* 18(6):859-867.

Wright, M.-O. 2008. Automated surveillance and infection control: Toward a better tomorrow. *American Journal of Infection Control* 36(3 Suppl 1):S1-S6.

Zhou, Y. Y., R. Unitan, J. J. Wang, T. Garrido, H. L. Chin, M. C. Turley, and L. Radler. 2011. Improving population care with an integrated electronic panel support tool. *Population Health Management* 14(1):3-9.

3

Examination of the Current State of the Art in System Safety and Its Relationship to the Safety of Health IT–Assisted Care

To understand the complex relationship of implementation and safety, this chapter presents key concepts of system safety and applies those concepts to the domains of health IT and patient safety.

SAFETY IN COMPLEX SYSTEMS

Complex systems are in general more difficult to operate and use safely than simple systems—with more components and more interfaces, there are a larger number of ways for untoward events to happen. Safety of complex systems in a variety of industries, such as health care (IOM, 2001), aviation (Orasanu et al., 2002), oil (Baker, 2007), and military operations (Snook, 2002), has been the focus of substantial research, and a number of broad lessons have emerged from this research.

Safety is a characteristic of a system—it is the product of its constituent components and their interaction. That is, safety is an emergent property of systems, especially complex systems. Failure in complex systems usually arises from multiple factors, not just one. The reason is that the designers and operators of complex systems are generally cognizant of the possibilities for failure, and thus over time they develop a variety of safeguards against failure (e.g., backup systems, safety features in equipment, safety training and procedures for operators). Such safeguards are most often useful in guarding against single-point failures, but it is often difficult to anticipate combinations of small failures that may lead to large ones. Put differently, the complexity of a system can mask interactions that could lead to systemic failure.

Nevertheless, complex systems often operate for extended periods of time without displaying catastrophic system-level failures. This is the result of good design as well as adaptation and intervention by those who operate and use the system on a routine basis. Extended failure-free operation is partially predicated on the ability of a complex system to adapt to unanticipated combinations of small failures (i.e., failures at the component level) and to prevent larger failures from occurring (i.e., failure of the entire system to perform its intended function). This adaptive capability is a product of both adherence to sound design principles and of skilled human operators who can react to avert system-level failure. In many cases, adaptations require human operators to select a well-practiced routine from a set of known and available responses. In some cases, adaptations require human operators to create on-the-fly novel combinations of known responses or de novo creations of new approaches to avert failures that result from good design or adaptation and intervention by those who use the system on a routine basis.

System safety is predicated on the affordances available to humans to monitor, evaluate, anticipate, and react to threats and on the capabilities of the individuals themselves. It should be noted that human operators (both individually and collectively as part of a team) serve in two roles: (1) as causes of and defenders against failure and (2) as producers of output (e.g., health care, power, transportation services). Before a system-wide failure, organizations that do not have a strong safety- and reliability-based culture tend to focus on their role as producers of output. However, when these same organizations investigate system-wide failures, they tend to focus on their role as defenders against failure. In practice, human operators must serve both roles simultaneously—and thus must find ways to appropriately balance these roles. For example, human operators may take actions to reduce exposure to the consequences of component-level failures, they may concentrate resources where they are most likely to be needed, and they may develop contingency plans for handling expected and unexpected failures.

When system-level failure does occur, it is almost always because the system does not have the capability to anticipate and adapt to unforeseen combinations of component failure, in addition to not having the ability to detect unforeseen adverse events early enough to mitigate their impact. By most measures, systems involving health IT are complex systems.

One fundamental reason for the complexity of systems involving health IT is that modern medicine is increasingly dependent on information—patient-specific information (e.g., symptoms, genomic information), general biomedical knowledge (e.g., diagnoses, treatments), and information related to an increasingly complex delivery system (e.g., rules, regulations, policies). The information of modern medicine is both large in volume and highly heterogeneous.

A second reason for the complexity of systems involving health IT is the large number of interacting actors who must work effectively with the information. For example, the provision of health care requires primary care physicians, nurses, physician and nurse specialists, physician extenders, health care payers, administrators, and allied health professionals, many of whom work in both inpatient and outpatient settings.

The IT needed to store, manage, analyze, and display large amounts of heterogeneous information for a wide variety and number of users is necessarily complex. Put differently, the complexity of health IT fundamentally reflects the complexity of medicine. Safety issues in health IT are largely driven by that complexity and the failure to proactively take appropriate systems-based action at all stages of the design, development, deployment, and operation of health IT.

THE NOTION OF A SOCIOTECHNICAL SYSTEM

The sociotechnical perspective takes the approach that the system is more than just the technology delivered to the user. The overall system—the sociotechnical system—consists of many components whose interaction with each other produces or accounts for the system's behavior (Fox, 1995). A sociotechnical view of health IT–assisted care might be depicted as in Figure 3-1.

For purposes of this report, the components of any sociotechnical system include the following:

- *Technology* includes the hardware and software of health IT, which are organized and developed under an architecture that specifies and delivers the functionality required from different parts of health IT, as well as how these different parts interact with each other. From the perspective of health professionals, technology can also include more clinically based information (e.g., order sets), although technologists regard order sets as the responsibility of clinical experts.
- *People* relates to individuals working within the entire sociotechnical system and includes their knowledge and skills regarding both clinical work and technology as well as their cognitive capabilities such as memory, inferential strategies, and knowledge. The "people" component also includes the implementation teams that configure and support the technology and those who train clinical users. People are affected by technology—for example, the use of health IT may affect clinician cognition by changing and shaping how clinicians obtain, organize, and reason with knowl-

People

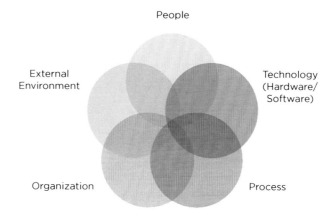

External
Environment

Technology
(Hardware/
Software)

Organization

Process

FIGURE 3-1
Sociotechnical system underlying health IT-related adverse events.

SOURCE: Adapted from Harrington et al. (2010), Sittig and Singh (2010),
and Walker et al. (2008).

edge.[1] The way knowledge of health care is organized makes a difference in how people solve problems. Clinicians' interactions with the technology and with each other in a technology-mediated fashion—both the scope and nature of these interactions—are very likely to affect clinical outcomes.

- *Process* (sometimes referred to as "workflow") refers to the normative set of actions and procedures clinicians are expected to perform during the course of delivering health care. Many of the procedures clinicians use to interact with the technology are prescribed, either formally in documentation (e.g., a user's manual) or informally by the norms and practices of the work environment immediately surrounding the individual. Process also includes tasks such as patient scheduling.

- *Organization* refers to how the organization installs health IT, makes configuration choices, and specifies interfaces with health

---

[1] As one illustration, the introduction of a computer-based patient record into a diabetes clinic was associated with changes in the strategies used by physicians for information gathering and reasoning. Differences between paper records and computer records were also found regarding the content and organization of information, with paper records having a narrative structure while the computer-based records were organized into discrete items of information. The differences in knowledge organization had an effect on data-gathering strategies, where the nature of doctor–patient dialogue was influenced by the structure of the computer-based patient record system (Patel et al., 2000).

IT products. Organizations also choose the appropriate clinical content to use. These choices reflect the organizational goals such as maximizing usage of expensive clinical facilities (e.g., computed tomography scanners, radiation therapy machines) and minimizing costs. Of particular relevance to this report is the organization's role in promoting the safety of patient care while maximizing effectiveness and efficiency. Organization also includes the rules and regulations set by individual institutions, such as hospital guidelines for treatment procedures that clinicians must follow, and the environment in which clinicians work. In many institutions, the environment of care is chaotic and unpredictable—many clinicians are often interrupted in the course of their day, subject to multiple distractions from patients and coworkers.

- *External environment* refers to the environment in which health care organizations operate. Essential aspects of the environment are the regulations that may originate with federal or state authorities or with private-sector entities such as accreditation organizations. For example, health care organizations are often required to publicly report errors made in the course of providing care at a variety of levels, including the private-sector, federal, and state levels.

A comprehensive analysis of the safety afforded by any given health care organization requires consideration of all of these domains taken as a whole and how they affect each other, that is, of the entire sociotechnical system.[2] For example, an organization may develop formal policies regarding workflow. In the interests of saving time and increasing productivity, health care professionals may modify the prescribed workflow or approved practices in ways of which organizational leadership may be unaware. Workflow also can affect patient care, as in cases in which psychiatric patients in the emergency room are transferred from a psychiatric unit to a general medical unit. Units are often specialized to accommodate the needs of a particular group of patients; thus, the transfer of a psychiatric patient to the medical section may result in suboptimal or even inappropriate care for his medical condition (e.g., a medication associated with substance withdrawal not prescribed, or monitoring for withdrawal not performed) (Cohen et al., 2007).

SAFETY AS A SYSTEM PROPERTY

A traditional perspective on technology draws a sharp distinction between technology and human users of the technology. The contrast between

---

[2] A conceptual model of some of the unintended consequences of information technologies in health care can be found in Harrison et al. (2007).

a traditional perspective of technology and the sociotechnical perspective has many implications for how to conceptualize safety in health IT–assisted care. Perhaps most important, in the traditional perspective, health IT–related adverse events are generally not recognized as systemic problems, that is, as problems whose causation or presence is influenced by all parts of the sociotechnical system (see Box 3-1).

From a traditional perspective, software failures are primarily the result of errors in the code causing the software to behave in a manner inconsistent with its performance requirements. All other errors are considered "human error." However, software-related safety problems can often arise as a misunderstanding of what the software should do to help clinicians accomplish their work. The representative of an electronic health record (EHR) vendor testified to the committee that a user error occurs when

---

BOX 3-1
Mismanaging Potassium Chloride (KCl) Levels
Part I: A Sociotechnical View

As a result of multiple medication errors, an elderly patient who was originally hypokalemic (suffering from low levels of KCl) became severely hyperkalemic (suffering from high levels of KCl). To treat the original hypokalemia, the diagnosing physician used the hospital's computerized provider order entry (CPOE) system to prescribe KCl to the patient. Although she used the coded entry fields to write the order, she also tried to limit the dose by communicating to the nurse the volume of KCl that should be administered because the CPOE system was not designed to recognize instructions written in comment boxes. However, the nurse either misinterpreted the note or did not read it and the patient received more KCl than the diagnosing physician intended. A second physician, not having been informed that the patient was already prescribed KCl, used the CPOE system to prescribe even more KCl to the patient. As a result of these and other errors, the patient became hyperkalemic (Horsky et al., 2005).

Here, the patient's hyperkalemia was not a result of any coding errors in the CPOE system. However, when the CPOE system was closely scrutinized, it was discovered that the interface's poor design (see Box 3-2) and failure to display important lab reports and medication history (see Box 3-3) were also major contributors to the patient's hyperkalemia. The patient's hyperkalemia was not solely caused by human or computer error. Instead, it was the result of combined interactions of poor technology, procedures, and people. The boxes throughout this chapter examine how these interactions all contributed to the hyperkalemia suffered by the patient.

a human takes some action under a certain set of circumstances that is inconsistent with the action prescribed in the software's documentation.[3] In this view, the software works as designed and the user makes an error. However, such views can have negative consequences. In examining the traditional perspective, a National Research Council report (NRC, 2007) concluded that:

> As is well known to software engineers (but not to the general public), by far the largest class of problems arises from errors made in the eliciting, recording, and analysis of requirements. A second large class of problems arises from poor human factors design. The two classes are related; bad user interfaces usually reflect an inadequate understanding of the user's domain and the absence of a coherent and well-articulated conceptual model.

By blaming users for making a mistake and not considering poor human factors design, the organization accepts responsibility only for training the individual user to do better the next time similar circumstances arise. But the overall system and the interactions among system components that might have led to the problem remain unexamined. Better training of users is important but it does not by itself address issues arising because of the overall system's operation. Other parts of the sociotechnical system—such as organization, technology, and processes—could also have increased the likelihood of an error occurring (see Box 3-2). Of particular importance to technology vendors is that adopting this unsophisticated oversimplification that user error is the principal actionable cause essentially exonerates any technology that may be involved. If the problem arises because the user failed to act in accordance with the technology's documentation, then it is the clinician's organization that must take responsibility for the problem, and vendors may feel that they need not take responsibility for making fixes for other users that may encounter a similar situation or for improving the technology to make serious errors less likely.

Applying the concept of the sociotechnical system of which technology is a part, safety is a property of the overall system that emerges from the interaction between its various components. By itself, software—such as an EHR—is neither safe nor unsafe; what counts from a safety perspective is how it behaves when in actual clinical use.

By viewing technology as part of a sociotechnical system, a number of realizations can be made. First, although individual components

---

[3] Testimony on February 24, 2011, to the committee by a health IT vendor defining "user error."

BOX 3-2
Mismanaging Potassium Chloride (KCl) Levels
Part II: Medication Errors Can Result from Poor Design

Although the physician in Box 3-1 typed instructions as free text, the physician had also attempted to use the computerized provider order entry (CPOE) system's coded order entry fields. However, the user interface design made it difficult to correctly write the orders. The CPOE system allowed KCl to be prescribed either by the length of time KCl is administered through an intravenous (IV) drip or by dosage through an IV injection. The CPOE system's interface headings, denoting the two types of orders, were subtle and hard to see; therefore, the physician may have been confused as to whether she should place her KCl IV drip order by volume or by time. Further complicating matters, a coded entry field for drip orders was labeled "Total Volume," which the physician may have interpreted as the total volume of fluid the patient will receive. However, the "Total Volume" field is meant to indicate the size of the IV drip bags (Horsky et al., 2005).

Here, instead of the CPOE system assisting the clinician in calculating the correct dosages, the system's poorly designed interface serves as a hindrance and increases the cognitive workload placed on clinicians. The CPOE system's design made it easy for clinicians to make a mistake. Vendors may claim that the software worked as designed and that clinicians should be better trained to use the design. However, it may be much more effective to appropriately design and simplify the CPOE system than to train all the clinicians to use a needlessly complicated system that requires an increased cognitive workload and is prone to misinterpretations. A safer system would be designed to make it difficult for a clinician to make a mistake that could result in harm to the patient.

of a system can be highly reliable,[4] the system as a whole can still yield unsafe outcomes. Second, while no component of any system is perfect or 100 percent reliable, even "unreliable" components can be assembled into a system that operates at an acceptable level of reliability at the systems level even in the face of individual system element failures. Third, the distinction between "human error" and "computer error" is misleading. Human errors should be seen as the result of human variability, which is an integral element in human learning and adaptation (Rasmussen, 1985). This approach considers the human–task or human–machine mismatches

---

[4] Reliability is used here as behavior that is consistent with the stated performance requirements of those components. Reliability does not speak to whether those stated requirements are correct.

as a basis for analysis and classification of human errors, instead of solely tasks or machines (Rasmussen et al., 1987). These mismatches could also stem from inappropriate work conditions, lack of familiarity, or improper (human–machine) interface design.

From the sociotechnical perspective, safety issues commonly arise from how practitioners interact with the technology in question. "Human error" in using technology can be more properly regarded as an inconsistency between the user's expectations about how the system will behave and the assumptions made by technology designers about how the system should behave. In some cases, the system is designed in a way that induces human behavior, resulting in unsafe system behavior. Human behavior is a product of the environment in which it occurs; to reduce or to manage human error, the environment in which the human works must be changed (Leveson, 2009). This implies thoughtful design that can proactively mitigate the risk of harm when health IT is used.

Finally, when complex systems are involved, a superficial event-chain model of an unsafe event is inadequate for understanding such events but is often employed by unsophisticated organizations. This model is described in terms of event A (the unsafe event) being caused by event B (the "proximate cause"), which was caused by event C, and so on until the "root cause" is identified.

Many problematic events involving complex systems cannot be ascribed to a single causative factor. Although the model described above provides some information as to the cause, it fails to account both for the conditions that allowed the preceding events to occur and for the indirect, usually systemic factors that increase the likelihood of these conditions occurring. Furthermore, because the decision to terminate the chain at any given event is essentially arbitrary, the single root cause is frequently ascribed to human error, as though possible system-induced causes of human error need not be further investigated. Investigations that find human error to be the root cause, while common, are usually inadequate and result in corrective action that essentially directs people to be "more careful" rather than to examine the constellation of contributing factors that make a so-called human error more likely (see Box 3-3).

The primary lesson from this perspective on safety can be described as the following: "Task analysis focused on action sequences and occasional deviation in terms of human errors should be replaced by a model of behavior-shaping mechanisms in terms of work system constraints, boundaries of acceptable performance, and subjective criteria guiding adaptation to change" (Rasmussen, 1997).

BOX 3-3
Mismanaging Potassium Chloride (KCl) Levels
Part III: Medication Errors Caused by Multiple Factors

After receiving an excessive amount of KCl by the diagnosing physician, the patient described in Box 3-1 was prescribed an additional dose of KCl by a second physician. Although told by the first physician to review the patient's KCl levels, the second physician was unaware that the patient was already being administered an excessive amount of KCl due to several factors. These factors included the following:

1. The previous physician did not explicitly inform the second physician that KCl was already ordered.
2. The KCl IV drip did not appear in the computerized provider order entry (CPOE) system's medication list because IV drips are not displayed in the CPOE's medication list.
3. The CPOE only showed the patient's lab results before the administration of the KCl drip ordered by the first physician; therefore, the second physician only saw the patient's previously low levels of KCl (Horsky et al., 2005).

Although the second physician had checked the previous physician's notes, medication history, and lab reports, there was no indication that the patient was already receiving KCl. These factors, including the poorly designed CPOE interface, may not be identified in a single event chain, yet each independently contributed to the patient's excessive KCl levels. Looking for a single "root cause" responsible for the patient's adverse condition would fail to address the other factors that may continue to put future patients at risk.

THE NEED FOR AN EXPLICIT
EVIDENCE-BASED CASE FOR SAFETY IN SOFTWARE[5]

Safety has no useful meaning for software until a clear understanding is achieved regarding what the software should and should not do and under what circumstances these things do and do not happen. (In this context, safety refers to claimed properties of software that make it safe enough to use for its intended purpose.)

When safety is at issue, the burden of proof falls on the software developer to make a convincing case that the software is safe enough for use. The audience for the case differs depending on the situation at hand.

---

[5] This section is based in large part on *Software for Dependable Systems* (NRC, 2007).

For example, it may be the software vendor who must make the safety case to a prospective purchaser of its products, or to an entity that might provide a safety certification for a given product. Once the software has been developed, installed, and the relevant processes and procedures put into place for proper software use, it may be the health care organization that must make the safety case for the overall system—that is, the software as installed into a larger sociotechnical system—to an external oversight organization responsible for ensuring the safe operation of care providers.

Such a case cannot be made by relying primarily on adherence to particular software development processes, although such adherence may be part of a case for safety. Nor can the safety case be made by relying primarily on a thorough testing regimen. Rigorous development and testing processes are critical elements of software safety, but they are not sufficient to demonstrate it. Developing a comprehensive case for safety that can be independently assessed depends on the generation, availability, communicability, and clarity of evidence. Three elements are necessary to develop a case for safety:

- *Explicit claims of safety.* No software is safe in all respects and under all conditions. Thus, to claim software is safe, an explicit articulation is needed of the requirements and properties the software is expected to possess and exhibit in use and the assumptions about the environment in which the software operates and usage models upon which such a claim is contingent. Explicit claims of safety further depend on the inclusion of a hazard analysis. Hazard analyses ought to identify and assess potential hazards and the conditions that can lead to them so that they can be eliminated or controlled (Leveson, 1995).

- *Evidence.* A case for safety must argue that the required behavioral properties of the software are a consequence of the combination of the actual technology involved (that is, as implemented), users, the processes and procedures they use, and other aspects of the larger sociotechnical system within which the technology is embedded. All domains of the sociotechnical system must be taken into account in the development of a case for safety. Evidence acquired from testing the software will be part of this case, but "lab" testing alone is usually insufficient. The case for software safety typically combines evidence from testing with evidence from analysis. Other evidence also contributes to the safety case, including the qualifications of the personnel involved in the system's development, the safety and quality track record of the organizations in building the system's components, integration of the components into the overall system, and the process through which the software was developed. Furthermore, the safety case must present evidence that

use of the technology in the actual work environment by real clinicians with real patients demonstrates functioning without a level of
malfunction greater than that specified in the design requirements.
- *Expertise.* Expertise—in software development and in the relevant
  clinical domains, among other things—is necessary to build safe
  software. Furthermore, those with expertise in these different contexts must communicate effectively with each other and be involved
  at every step of the design, development, and component integration process.

When software is complex, it can be difficult to determine its safety
properties. An analytical argument for safety is easier to make when global
safety properties of the software can be inferred from an analysis of the
safety properties of its components. Such inferences are more likely to be
possible when different parts of the system are designed to operate independently of each other.

Achieving simplicity is not easy or cheap, but simpler software is much
easier for independent assessors to evaluate, and the rewards of simplicity
far outweigh its costs (NRC, 2007). Pitfalls to avoid include interactive
complexity, in which components may interact in unanticipated ways and
a single fault cannot be isolated but it causes other faults that cascade
through the software. Avoiding these characteristics both reduces the likelihood of failure and simplifies the safety case to be made.

Most important to developing a plausible case for safety is the stance
that developers take toward safety. A developer is better able to make a
plausible safety case when it is willing to provide safety-related data from
all phases in the components' or software's life cycle, to ensure the clarity and integrity of the data provided and the coherence of the safety case
made, and to accept responsibility for safety failures. One report goes so
far as to assert that "no software should be considered dependable if it is
supplied with a disclaimer that withholds the manufacturer's commitment
to provide a warranty or other remedies for software that fails to meet its
dependability claims" (NRC, 2007).

With respect to health IT, it is not often that health care organizations
make an explicit case for the safety of health IT in situ, and not often that
vendors make an explicit case for the safety of their health IT products.

THE (MIS)MATCH BETWEEN THE ASSUMPTIONS OF SOFTWARE DESIGNERS AND THE ACTUAL WORK ENVIRONMENT

Generally, health IT software is created by professionals in software
development, not by clinicians as content experts. Content experts are
usually provided with multiple opportunities to offer input into the perfor-

mance requirements that the software must meet (e.g., users brief software developers on how they perform various tasks and what they need the software to do, and they have opportunities to provide feedback on prototypes before designs are finalized). Traditionally, technology development follows a process where users of the technology articulate their needs (or performance requirements) to developers. Developers create technology that performs in accordance with their understanding of user needs. Users then test the resulting technology and provide feedback to developers. Developers provide a new version that incorporates that feedback and, when users are satisfied with the technology, the developer assumes it is suitable for use in the user's environment and delivers the technology. However, software developers and clinicians generally come from different backgrounds, making communication of ideas more difficult. As a result, these processes for gaining input rarely capture the full richness and complexity of the actual operational environment in which health professionals work and vary enormously from setting to setting and practitioner to practitioner.[6]

Deviations Versus Adherence to Formal Procedures

Indeed, in most organizations, guidance provided by formal procedures is rarely followed exactly by health professionals. Although this lack of user predictability can dramatically increase the difficulty for the software developer to deliver the degree of functional robustness required, deviations between work-as-designed and work-in-practice (work-in-practice is sometimes regarded as a workaround) are not necessarily harmful or negative. Such deviations are necessary under circumstances not anticipated by rules governing work-as-designed. In some cases, deviations are necessary if work is to be performed at all (Kahol et al., 2011).

Deliberate deviations between work-as-designed and work-in-practice are smallest when significant changes are made to the work environment— and the introduction of new technology usually counts as a significant change. Deviations are smallest during this period of introduction because practitioners are unfamiliar with the new technology and are learning about its capabilities for the first time. But, as practitioners become more familiar with the new technology, the limitations imposed by the new technology become more apparent in the local work environment. Practitioners thus develop modified—possibly unsanctioned—practices for using the technol-

---

[6] For example, Suchman (1987) argues that user actions depend on a variety of circumstances that are not explicitly related to the task at hand. In practice, the behavior of people varies if they are in the presence of other people (when they can ask for advice about what actions to take), for example if they are unusually pressed for time (in which case they may take possibly risky shortcuts).

ogy that account for the on-the-ground requirements of doing work; this process is sometimes known as "drift" (Snook, 2002) or workarounds and reflects the phenomenon of local rationality in which practitioners are all doing reasonable things given their limited perspective but the modified practices result in poor outcomes (Woods et al., 2010).

Sometimes modified practices are needed to manage conflicting goals that arise in an operational environment (e.g., pressures for speedy resolution versus pressures for collecting more data) (Woods et al., 2010). Under some circumstances, adherence to prescribed procedures can indeed result in unsafe outcomes. Although modified practices may be required to make the overall system safer, the modified practices themselves can sometimes result in unsafe outcomes. Almost by definition, the situations for which the use of the modified practices is unsafe occur only rarely. Practitioners adopt the modified practices to cope more effectively with frequently occurring situations, but the modified practices have mostly not been developed with the rarely occurring situation in mind.

Herein lies a critical safety paradox. Practitioners following the prescribed procedures may be unable to complete all of their work, which may motivate them to use nonstandard or unapproved approaches. If a disaster occurs because they did not follow the prescribed procedures in a given instance, they may be blamed for not following procedures. As discussed previously, unsafe outcomes result not from human failures per se but rather from the way the various components of the larger sociotechnical system interact with each other.

Clumsy Automation

A particularly relevant illustration of mismatches between the assumptions of software designers and the actual work environment can be seen in the notion of clumsy automation (Woods et al., 2010). Clumsy automation "creates additional tasks, forces the user to adopt new cognitive strategies, [and] requires more knowledge and more communication at the very times when the practitioners are most in need of true assistance" (see Box 3-4). At such times, practitioners can least afford to spawn new tasks and meet new memory demands to fiddle with the technology, and such results "create opportunities for new kinds of human error and new paths to system breakdown that did not exist in simpler systems" (Woods et al., 2010).

Clumsy automation reflects poor coordination between human users and information technology. Even clumsy automation often offers benefits when user workload is low (which is why systems that offer clumsy automation are so often accepted initially), but the costs and burdens of such automation become most apparent during periods of high workload, high criticality, or high-tempo operations.

BOX 3-4
Mismanaging Potassium Chloride (KCl) Levels
Part IV: Poor Performance Due to Clumsy Automation

The computerized provider order entry (CPOE) interface described in Box 3-1 did not have one screen that lists previous medication and drip orders, up-to-date laboratory results, or whether the patient is currently receiving a KCl drip (Horsky et al., 2005). Here, clinicians may need to switch between different display windows to ascertain all the information needed to complete KCl calculations. This requires the practitioner to enter keying sequences that are quite arbitrary and to remember what was on previous screens as he switches between them. The practitioner becomes the de facto integrating agent for all such data and hence bears the brunt of all the cognitive demands required for such integration (Woods et al., 2010). Furthermore, practitioners who work in a chaotic interruption-driven environment must turn their efforts to many other tasks before they have completed the task on which they are currently working. In such an inadequately designed environment, it is easy for a practitioner to lose context, to get lost in a multitude of windows, and to regain context of the interrupted task only partially, resulting in a higher risk of patient harm.

The use of a computerized interface—usually a video display screen—to display data can provide examples of the phenomenon of clumsy automation. Poorly designed computerized interfaces tend to make interesting and noteworthy things invisible when they hide important data behind a number of windows on the screen (Woods et al., 2010). Thus, practitioners are forced to access data serially even when the data are highly related and are most usefully viewed in parallel.

SAFETY REPORTING AND IMPROVEMENT

The safety of a system may degrade over time if attention is not given to ensuring system safety. Over time, technology changes as fixes and upgrades are made to the applications and the infrastructure on which those applications run, and the changes may often not be systems based and may be made without considering their impact on operational tasks. Experienced personnel depart and inexperienced personnel arrive. External regulations and institutional priorities both evolve, and thus operating procedures change.

When such changes are large, they are often accompanied by formal documentation that modifies existing work-as-designed procedures. But more often, changes to work-in-practice occur with little formal documentation. As the system's work-in-practice drifts farther away from work-as-designed, the likelihood of certain unsafe outcomes increases, as discussed above. For this reason, safety-conscious overseers of the system will audit the system from time to time so that they can identify budding safety problems and take action to forestall them.

But it is hard to know where to look for problems in a system that appears to be performing safely. Thus, all parties responsible for safety must make it easy for practitioners to report circumstances that result in actual harm and also to report close calls that could have resulted in harm if they had not been caught in time.

In addition, because the society in which the U.S. health care system is embedded (that is, society writ large) generally seeks to apportion responsibility and fault for actual harm, health professionals—who are in the best position to know what actually happened in any given accident—often have incentives to refrain from reporting fully or at all when unsafe conditions occur. Thus, information that is needed to improve the safety of health care—and of health IT–assisted care in particular—is likely to be systematically suppressed and underreported. Reporting mechanisms must therefore be structured to offer countervailing incentives for such reporting. Safety analysts often point to the "Just Culture" principles for dealing with incident reporting (Global Aviation Information Network Working Group E, 2004; Marx, 2001; Reason, 1997). Based on the notion that the safety afforded by an organization can benefit more by learning from mistakes than by punishing people who make them, a Just Culture organization encourages people to report errors and to suggest changes as part of their normal everyday duties. People can report without jeopardy, and mistakes or incidents are seen not as failure but as an opportunity to focus attention and to learn. Thus, information provided in good faith is not used against those who report it.

The Just Culture organization recognizes that most people are genuinely concerned for the safety of their work, and it takes advantage of the fact that when reporting of problems leads to visible improvements, employees need few other motivations or exhortations to report. In Leveson's words, "empowering people to affect their work conditions and making the reporters of safety problems part of the change process promotes their willingness to shoulder their responsibilities and to share information about safety problems. . . . Blame is the enemy of safety . . . [and] when blame is a primary component of the safety culture, people stop reporting incidents" (Leveson, 2009).

CONCLUSION

The idea that safety is an emergent property of a sociotechnical system is easy to acknowledge in the abstract. But in fact, the implications of taking such a view challenges many widespread practices found in health IT vendors and health care–providing organizations. Vendors often focus on the role of technology when safety is compromised, and they pledge to fix any technology problems thus found without addressing the human-interaction component in the overall functioning of the technology as an inextricable component of health IT as a clinical tool. Because complex systems almost always fail in complex ways (a point noted in safety examinations in other fields[7]), health care organizations must focus on identifying the conditions and factors that contribute to safety compromises. They must pledge to address these conditions and factors in ways that reduce the likelihood of unsafe events rather than superficially focusing only on single root causes. Failure to acknowledge that technology-related problems that are encountered are a product of larger systems-based issues will result in the implementation of countermeasures that will fall far short with regard to the reduction of risk to the patient.

The fact that a sociotechnical system has multiple components that interact with each other in unpredictable ways means that an isolated examination of any one of these components will not yield many reliable insights into the behavior of the examined component as it operates in actual practice. This point has implications for technology developers in particular, who must develop products that can fit well into the operational practices and workflow (which are usually nonlinear) of many different health care organizations. The next chapter suggests various levers with which to improve safety.

REFERENCES

Baker, J. A. 2007. *The report of the BP U.S. Refineries Independent Safety Review Panel.* http://www.bp.com/liveassets/bp_internet/globalbp/globalbp_uk_english/SP/STAGING/local_assets/assets/pdfs/Baker_panel_report.pdf (accessed September 28, 2011).

Cohen, T., B. Blatter, C. Almeida, and V. L. Patel. 2007. Reevaluating recovery: Perceived violations and preemptive interventions on emergency psychiatry rounds. *Journal of the American Medical Informatics Association* 14(3):312-319.

Fox, W. M. 1995. Sociotechnical system principles and guidelines: Past and present. *Journal of Applied Behavioral Science* 31(1):91-105.

Global Aviation Information Network Working Group E. 2004. *A roadmap to a just culture: Enhancing the safety environment.* http://204.108.6.79/products/documents/roadmap%20to%20a%20just%20culture.pdf (accessed August 9, 2011).

Harrison, M. I., R. Koppel, and S. Bar-Lev. 2007. Unintended consequences of information technologies in health care—an interactive sociotechnical analysis. *Journal of the American Medical Informatics Association* 14(5):542-549.

---

[7] This point was noted in the report of the Board investigating the Shuttle Columbia disaster (http://spaceflightnow.com/columbia/report/006boardstatement.html) and in the investigation of the Deepwater oil rig explosion (http://www.deepwaterinvestigation.com/go/doc/3043/1193483/).

Horsky, J., G. J. Kuperman, and V. L. Patel. 2005. Comprehensive analysis of a medication dosing error related to CPOE. *Journal of the American Medical Informatics Association* 12(4):377-382.

IOM (Institute of Medicine). 2001. *Crossing the quality chasm: A new health system for the 21st century*. Washington, DC: National Academy Press.

Kahol, K., M. Vankipuram, V. L. Patel, and M. L. Smith. 2011. Deviations from protocol in a complex trauma environment: Errors or innovations? *Journal of Biomedical Informatics* 44(3):425-431.

Leveson, N. 1995. *Safeware: System safety and computers*. Reading, MA: Addison-Wesley.

Leveson, N. 2009. *Engineering a safer world: Systems thinking applied to safety*. http://sunnyday.mit.edu/safer-world/safer-world.pdf (accessed June 1, 2011).

Marx, D. 2001. *Patient safety and the "just culture": A primer for health care executives*. New York, NY: Columbia University. Available at http://psnet.ahrq.gov/resource.aspx?resourceID=1582.

NRC (National Research Council). 2007. *Software for dependable systems*. Washington, DC: The National Academies Press.

Orasanu, J., L. H. Martin, and J. Davison. 2002. Cognitive and contextual factors in aviation accidents: Decision errors. In *Linking expertise and naturalistic decision making*, edited by E. Salas and G. Klein. Mahwah, NJ: Erlbaum Associates. Pp. 209-226.

Patel, V. L., A. W. Kushniruk, S. Yang, and J.-F. Yale. 2000. Impact of a computer-based patient record system on data collection, knowledge organization, and reasoning. *Journal of the American Medical Informatics Association* 7(6):569-585.

Rasmussen, J. 1985. Trends in human reliability analysis. *Ergonomics* 28(8):1185-1195.

Rasmussen, J. 1997. Risk management in a dynamic society: A modelling problem. *Safety Science* 27(2-3):183-213.

Rasmussen, J., K. Duncan, and J. Leplat. 1987. *New technology and human error*. New York: John Wiley & Sons.

Reason, J. 1997. *Managing the risks of organizational accidents*. Hants, England: Ashgate.

Snook, S. A. 2002. *Friendly fire: The accidental shootdown of U.S. Blackhawks over northern Iraq*. Princeton, NJ: Princton University Press.

Suchman, L. 1987. *Plans and situated actions: The problem of human machine communication*. New York: Cambridge University Press.

Woods, D., S. Dekker, R. Cook, L. Johannesen, and N. Sarter. 2010. *Behind human error*, 2nd ed. Burlington, VT: Ashgate.

4

Opportunities to Build a Safer System for Health IT

Health IT supports a safety-critical system: its design, implementation, and use can either provide a substantial improvement in the quality and safety of patient care or pose serious risks to patients. In any sociotechnical system, consideration of the interactions of the people, processes, and technology form the baseline for ensuring successful system performance. Evidence suggests that existing health IT products in actual use may not yet be consistently producing the anticipated benefits, indicating that health IT products, in some cases, can contribute to unintended risks of harm.

To improve safety, health IT needs to optimize the interaction between people, technology, and the rest of the sociotechnical system. Sociotechnical theory, as described in Chapter 3, advocates for direct involvement of end users in system design. It shifts the paradigm for software development from technical development done in isolation by software and systems engineers to a process that is inclusive and iterative, engaging end users in design, deployment, and integration of the software product into workflow to enhance satisfaction and effectiveness.

Adhering to well-developed practices for design, training, and use can minimize safety risks. Building safer health IT involves exploring both real and potential hazards so that hazards are minimized or eliminated. Health IT can be viewed as having two related but distinct life cycles, with one relating to the design and development of health IT and the other associated with the implementation and use of health IT. Vendors and implementing organizations have specific roles in all phases of both life cycles and ought to coordinate their efforts for ensuring safety. The size, complexity, and resources available to large and small clinician practices and health care

77

organizations may affect their abilities to fully realize the benefits of health IT products intended to facilitate safer care. This chapter reflects as much as possible the literature, experiences of key stakeholders, and the committee's expert opinion.

FEATURES OF SAFE HEALTH IT

Technology does not exist in isolation from its operator. As such, the design and use of health IT are interdependent. The design and development of products affects their safe performance and the extent to which clinician users will accept or reject the technology. To the end user, a safely functioning health IT product is one that includes

- Easy retrieval of accurate, timely, and reliable native and imported data;
- A system the user wants to interact with;
- Simple and intuitive data displays;
- Easy navigation;
- Evidence at the point of care to aid decision making;
- Enhancements to workflow, automating mundane tasks, and streamlining work, never increasing physical or cognitive workload;
- Easy transfer of information to and from other organizations and providers; and
- No unanticipated downtime.

Investing in health IT products aims to make care safer and improve health professional workflow while not introducing harm or risks. Key features such as enhanced workflow, usability, balanced customization, and interoperability affect whether or not clinician users enjoy successful interactions with the product and achieve these aims. Effective design and development drive the safe functioning of the products as well as determine some aspects of safe use by health professionals. Collaboration among users and vendors across the continuum of technology design, including embedding products into clinical workflow and ongoing product optimization, represents a dynamic process characterized by frequent feedback and joint accountability to promote safer health IT. The combination of these activities can result in building safer systems for health IT, as summarized in Figure 4-1.

Safer Systems for Health IT Seamlessly Support Cognitive and Clinical Workflows

The cognitive work of clinicians is substantial. Clinicians must rapidly integrate large amounts of data to make decisions in unstable and complex

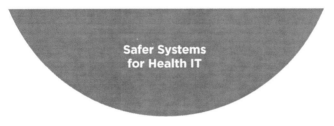

Health Professionals,
Health Care Organizations,
Vendors

Features of Health IT	Design and Development	Implementation
– Workflow	– Software requirements and development	– Planning and goal setting
– Usability	– User interface design	– Deployment
– Balanced customization	– Testing	– Stabilization
– Interoperability	– Deployment	– Optimization
	– Maintenance and upgrade	– Transformation

Safer Systems
for Health IT

FIGURE 4-1
Interdependent activities for building a safer system for health IT.

settings. The use of health IT is intended to aid in performing technical work that is also cognitive work, such as coordinating resources for a procedure, assembling patient data for action, or supporting a decision that requires knowledge of resource availability. However, creating a graphical representation of the information needed to support the complex processes clinicians use to collect and analyze data elements, consider alternative choices, and then make a definitive decision is challenging.

The introduction of health IT sometimes changes clinical workflows in unanticipated ways; these changes may be detrimental to patient safety. Although some templates may be very useful to providers, a rigid template for recording the "history of present illness," for example, may alter the conversation between physician and patient in such a way that important historical clues are not conveyed or received. An inflexible order sequence may require the provider to hold important orders in mind while navigating through mandatory screens, increasing the cognitive workload of communicating patient care orders and adding to the possibility that intended orders are forgotten. A time-consuming process for locating laboratory or radiographic data presents a barrier to retrieval. In addition, the time spent on cumbersome data retrieval and data remodeling is time taken away from other clinical demands, requiring shortcuts in other aspects of care. Evaluation of the impact of introducing health IT on the cognitive workload of clinicians is important to determine unintended consequences and the potential for distraction, delays in care, and increased workload in general.

The timeframe for greatest threats to safety is during initial implementation, when workflow is new, a steep learning curve threatens previous practice, and nonperformance of any aspect of a technology causes the user to seek immediate alternate pathways to achieve a particular functionality, otherwise called a workaround. Alternatively, users of mature health IT products are at risk for habituation and overreliance on a technology, requiring vigilant attention to alerts or other notifications so that safety features are not ignored. When use of health IT impedes workflow, there must be a way to identify not only the faulty process that results but also any potential increase in workload for clinicians.

Workarounds, common in health IT environments, are often a symptom of suboptimal design. When workarounds circumvent built-in safety features of a product, patient safety may be compromised. Integrating health IT within real-world clinical workflows requires attention to in situ use to ensure appropriate use of safety features (Koppel et al., 2008).

For example, coping mechanisms such as "paste forward" (or "copy forward"), a practice of copying portions of previously entered documentation and reusing the text in a new note, may be understood as compensatory survival strategies in an environment where the electronic environment does not support an efficient clinician workflow. However, this function may encourage staff to repeat an earlier evaluation rather than consider whether it is still accurate. In addition, the problem list in some electronic health records (EHRs) is limited to structured International Classification of Diseases (ninth revision) (ICD-9) entries, which may not capture the relevant clinical information required for optimal care. Paste forward is then employed as a means of bringing forward important, longitudinal data, such as richly detailed descriptions of the prior evaluation and medical thinking for each of a patient's multiple medical problems that otherwise is not accommodated in the EHR. Yet, if done without exquisite attention to detail, these workarounds themselves can create risk. The optimal design and implementation of EHRs should include a deep understanding of and response to the clinician-initiated workarounds.

Usability Is a Key Driver of Safety

Health professionals work in complex, high-risk, and frequently chaotic environments fraught with interruptions, time pressures, and incomplete, disorganized, and overwhelming amounts of information. Health professionals require technologies that make this work easier and safer, rather than more difficult. Health IT products are needed that promote efficiency and ease of use while minimizing the likelihood of error.

Many health information systems used today provide poor support for the cognitive tasks and workflow of clinicians (NRC, 2009). This can lead to clinicians spending time unnecessarily identifying the most relevant data for clinical decision making, potentially selecting the wrong data, and missing important information that may increase patient safety risks. If the design of the software disrupts an efficient workflow or presents a cumbersome user interface, the potential for harm rises (see Box 4-1). Software design and its effect on workflow, as well as an effective user interface, are key determinants of usability.

The committee expressed concerns that poor usability, such as the example in Box 4-1, is one of the single greatest threats to patient safety. On the other hand, once improved, it can be an effective promoter of patient safety.

The common expectation is that health IT should make "the right thing to do the easy thing to do" as facilitated by effective design. Evaluation of the impact of health IT on usability and on cognitive workload is important to determine unintended consequences and the potential for distraction, delays in care, and increased workload in general.

Usability guidelines and principles focused on improving safety need to be put into practice. Research over the past several decades supports a number of usability guidelines and principles. For example, there are a finite number of styles with which a user may interact with a computer system: direct manipulation (e.g., moving objects on a screen), menu selection, form fill-in, command language, and natural language. Each of these styles has known advantages and disadvantages, and one (or perhaps a blend of two or more) may well be more appropriate for a specific application from a usability standpoint.

The National Institute of Standards and Technology (NIST) has been developing guidelines and standards for usability design and evaluation. One report, *NIST Guide to the Processes Approach for Improving the Usability of Electronic Health Records*, introduces the basic concepts of usability, common principles of good usability design, methods for usability evaluation and improvement, processes of usability engineering, and the importance of organizational commitment to usability (NIST, 2010b). The second report, *Customized Common Industry Format Template for Elec-*

BOX 4-1
Opportunities for Unintended Consequences

Health IT that is not designed to facilitate common tasks can result in unintended consequences.

- The most common ordering sequence is frequently not the most prominent sequence presented to the clinician, increasing the chance of an inadvertent error. For example, in the hospital setting, where anticoagulation is being initiated or where patient characteristics are in flux, the required dose of Coumadin varies from day to day. When the selections for "__ mg of Coumadin daily" appear at the top of the list of choices, there is an increased chance clinicians will inadvertently select "5 mg of Coumadin daily" rather than scrolling down to the bottom of the page and finding "5 mg of Coumadin today." This design–workflow mismatch may result in patients receiving unintended Coumadin doses or similarly may affect other medications requiring daily dose adjustment.
- When a patient's medications are listed alphabetically or randomly rather than grouped by type, users are forced through several pages of medications and mentally knit together the therapeutic program for each individual condition. In this situation, the cognitive workload of understanding of the patient's diabetic regimen, for example, is made unnecessarily complex, and a clinician may easily miss one of the patient's five diabetic medications, scattered among the patient's 24 medications displayed across three different pages. Likewise, a patient's congestive heart failure medications may be dispersed across the same several pages, interspersed with medications for other conditions, again increasing the mental workload. In one example, "furosemide 80 mg q am" was toward the top of the list and then, separated by many intervening medications and on the next page, the clinician later found an entry for "furosemide 40 mg q pm." Such data disorganization contributes to the possibility of clinical error.

Even if clinicians are aware of these issues and become more diligent, health IT products that are not designed for users' needs create additional cognitive workload, which, over time, may cause the clinician to be more susceptible to making mistakes.

Personal communication, Christine A. Sinsky, August 11, 2011.

tronic Health Record Usability Testing, is not only a template for reporting usability evaluation but also a guideline for what and how usability evaluation should be conducted (NIST, 2010a). NIST released draft guidance on design evaluation and human user performance testing for usability issues related to patient safety, *Technical Evaluation, Testing and Evaluation of the Usability of Electronic Health Records*. NIST will publish its final guidance based on constructive technical feedback received during a public comment process for the draft report (NIST, 2011).

The National Center for Cognitive Informatics and Decision Making in Healthcare (NCCD) has developed the Rapid Usability Assessment process to assess the usability of EHRs on specific meaningful use objectives and to provide detailed and actionable feedback to vendors to help improve their systems. The Rapid Usability Assessment process is based on two established methodologies. The first is the use of well-established usability principles to identify usability problems that are targets for potential improvements (Neilson, 1994; Zhang et al., 2003). This evaluation is performed by usability experts. The usability problems identified in the process are documented, rated for severity by the experts, and communicated to the vendors.

The second phase of the Rapid Usability Assessment involves the use of a technique known as the "keystroke-level model" (Card et al., 1983; Kieras, unpublished). Using this method, it is possible to estimate the time and steps required to complete specific tasks. This method makes the assumption that an expert user would be using the system and therefore provides the optimal or fastest time to complete the task. The Rapid Usability Assessment uses a software tool, CogTool, to enhance the accuracy and reliability of the keystroke-level model (John et al., 2004). The program calculates the amount of time an expert user will use to complete the task and steps involved in that task. A confidential report is provided to participating vendors, which includes objective measures of the usability of the system, actionable results, and opportunities for further consultation with the usability evaluation team. It is important to note that although usability is integral to safe systems, sometimes safe practices require taking more time to perform a task to do it safely.

In addition to the Rapid Usability Assessment, the NCCD also developed a unified framework for EHR usability, called TURF, which stands for the four major factors for usability: task, user, representation, and function (Zhang and Walji, 2011). TURF is a theory that describes, explains, and predicts usability differences across EHR systems. It is also a framework that defines and measures EHR usability systematically and objectively. The NCCD is currently developing and testing software tools to automate a subset of the features of TURF, but these tests are still laboratory based.

A dynamic tension exists between the need for design standards development and vendor competitive differentiation, which is discussed further in the next section. As a result, dissemination of best practices for EHR design has been restrained (McDonnell et al., 2010). Without a comprehensive set of standards for EHR-specific functionalities, general software usability design practices are used knowing that modification will likely be needed to meet the needs of health professionals.

User-centered design and usability testing takes into account knowledge, preferences, workflow, and human factors associated with the complex information needs of varied providers in diverse settings. Many new product enhancements address functionalities desired by users that facilitate or improve workflow and improve on current health IT products. One such example is the electronic capture of gestures observed in an operating room that is then recorded as activities requiring no interruption of the clinician's working within the sterile field. To support usability within EHRs, Shneiderman has identified eight heuristically and experientially derived "golden rules" for interface design (Shneiderman et al., 2009) (see Table 4-1).

Achieving the Right Balance Between Customization and Standardization

Current health IT products do not arrive as finished products ready for out-of-the-box or turnkey deployment, but rather often require substantial completion on site. Many smaller organizations do not have the resources for such onsite "customization" and must get by without the products being user ready. For example, when a large institution recognized the need for a diabetic flow sheet that was not supplied by the vendor, it created its own diabetic flow sheet locally. A smaller organization, using the same EHR product and with the same need for a diabetic flow sheet, did not have this capability and its clinicians reverted to a paper workaround using a handwritten flow sheet.

Widespread institution-specific customization presents challenges to maintenance, upgrades, sharing of best practices, and interoperability across multiple-user organizations. Some standardization is necessary, but too much standardization can unnecessarily restrict an organization. In some instances, the implementing organization needs to customize and adapt innovation—the product being integrated—in order to better adopt the innovation (Berwick, 2003). The committee believes there is value in standardization and expressed the need for judicious use of customization when appropriate. Vendors are encouraged to provide more complete, responsive, and resilient health IT products as a preferred way to decrease the need for extensive customization.

TABLE 4-1
Eight Golden Rules for Interface Design

Principles	Characteristics

Strive for consistency	– Similar tasks ought to have similar sequences of action to perform, for example:
	  • Identical terminology in prompts and menus
	  • Consistent screen appearance
	– Any exceptions should be understandable and few

Cater to universal usability	– Users span a wide range of expertise and have different desires, for example:
	  • Expert users may want shortcuts
	  • Novices may want explanations

Offer informative feedback	– Systems should provide feedback for every user action to:
	  • Reassure the user that the appropriate action has been or is being done
	  • Instruct the user about the nature of an error if one has been made
	– Infrequent or major actions call for substantial responses, while frequent or minor actions require less feedback

Design dialogs to yield closure	– Have a beginning, middle, and end to action sequences – Provide informative feedback when a group of actions has been completed – Signal that it is okay to drop contingency plans – Indicate the need for preparing the next group of actions

Prevent errors	– Systems should be designed so that users cannot make serious errors, for example:
	  • Do not display menu items that are not appropriate in a given context
	  • Do not allow alphabetic characters in numeric entry fields
	– User errors should be detected and instructions for recovery offered
	– Errors should not change the system state

Permit easy reversal of actions	– When possible, actions (and sequences of actions) should be reversible
Support internal locus of control	– Surprises or changes should be avoided in familiar behaviors and complex data-entry sequences
Reduce short-term memory load	– Interfaces should be avoided if they require users to remember information from one screen for use in connection with another screen

Interoperability

Increased interoperability (i.e., the ability to exchange health information between health IT products and across organizational boundaries) can improve patient safety (Kaelber et al., 2008). Multiple levels of interoperability exist and are needed for different levels of communication (see Table 4-2). Currently, laboratory data have been relatively easy to exchange because good standards exist such as Logical Observation Identifiers Names and Codes (LOINC) and are widely accepted. However, important information such as problem lists and medication lists (which exist in some health IT products) are not easily transmitted and understood by the receiving health IT product because existing standards have not been uniformly adopted. Standards need to be further developed to support interoperability throughout all health IT products.

The committee believes interoperability must extend throughout the continuum of care, including pharmacies, laboratories, ambulatory, acute, post-acute, home, and long-term care settings. For all these organizations to safely coordinate care, health IT products must use common nomenclatures, encoding formats, and presentation formats. Interoperability with personal health record systems and other patient engagement tools is also desirable, both in delivering data to patients and in collecting information from any patient-operated systems.

Failure to achieve interoperability has considerable risks for patient safety. Without the ability of different health IT products to exchange data, information must be transferred by hand or electronic means outside the primary method (e.g., facsimile). Every time information is copied or transmitted by hand, there is a risk of error or loss of data. Incomplete and erroneous records may cause delays in care and result in harm.

Imported data must be timely, accurate, accessible, and displayed in a user-friendly fashion. Patient safety can be at risk even among products that have achieved some level of interoperability. For example, when a data value expected as a number arrives as a string, it can be misinterpreted, resulting in a wrong display. Also, electrocardiogram tracings can be displayed on a screen split in parts and rotated 90 degrees. The extra time required to mentally process such data into what is familiar delays care and increases the chance of error.

The nationwide exchange of data is intended to support portability and immediate access to one's health information. However, the competitive marketplace today provides few incentives for vendors themselves to support portability. The committee believes conformance tests ought to be available to clinicians so they can ensure their data are exchangeable. Independent entities need to be supported to develop "stress tests" that can be applied to validate whether medical record interoperability can be

TABLE 4-2
Aspects of Interoperability and Their Impact on Patient Safety

Aspects of Interoperability	Definition	Impact on Patient Safety
Ability to exchange the physical data stream of bits (Hoekstra et al., 2009) that represent relevant information	Allows for electronic communication between software components	Software components that cannot communicate with each other force users to reenter data manually, which: – Detracts from time better used attending to patient safety and – Increases opportunities to enter misinformation
Ability to exchange data without loss of semantic content	Ability for software system to properly work when modules from different vendors are "plugged in"	The loss of meaning in received data compromises patient safety
Accept "plug-ins" seamlessly	Semantic content refers to information that allows software to understand the electronic bits	– The inability to use multiple modules within one organization decreases the likelihood that users can provide their patient information to another health IT product – Lack of "plug-in" interoperability means that the user does not have the ability to select modules from multiple vendors that may perform a specific function more safely
Display similar information in the same way	– Different health IT products display similar information in similar ways – Systems are consistent in matters such as screen position of fields, color, and units	When information is displayed inconsistently across organizations, the user must reconcile the different representations of the information mentally, which: – Requires an increased cognitive effort that could be better used toward safe care and – Increases the chance that a user may make a mistake

achieved. These should impose requirements that will ensure both completeness of the record (e.g., a drug administration should include dosage and time) and interoperability (e.g., the drug name and units should be available and displayable by the receiving system). Suitable organizations to develop conformance tests might be entities such as the ECRI Institute or the Certification Commission for Healthcare Information Technology. Smaller clinics are in particular need of testing to ensure interoperability. Vendors could facilitate this process by publicly documenting their product and identifying the conformance tests they ran successfully.

Making data exchangeable is primarily the responsibility of the vendors who produce the code. The committee believes guidelines need to be developed to support safe interoperability (see Box 4-2).

Safety Considerations for EHR Implementation in Small Practices and Small Hospitals

In examining the current state of health IT, it is important to recognize that experiences often differ for care providers in small settings as compared to others. This difference is often not well captured in the literature

---

BOX 4-2
Potential Guidelines for Safe Interoperability

The committee believes guidelines for safe interoperability are needed, such as the following:

- All health IT products should be able to export data in structured and standard formats, ready for use in other modules or systems, without loss of semantic content.
- All health IT products should provide their documentation without a fee and in an easily read form. All products should publicize their adherence to relevant standards.
- All health IT products should be able to display imported data in a way compatible with data generated internally, so that users need not exert additional mental effort to deal with data arriving from other software packages.
- Use of standards for data representation should be strongly encouraged, as should support for both the completion of important standards still being developed, such as the RxNorm drug nomenclature effort at the National Library of Medicine, and the adoption of standards that exist but lack adequate adherence, such as SNOMED (Systematized Nomenclature for Medicine).

but instead recounted in personal experiences, which are the basis for this section. An emphasis on safety specific to small practices and hospitals—as well as rural providers and federal health centers—is particularly important because they provide a large fraction of the services delivered by the health care system.[1] These providers are often unfamiliar with system safety as an office concept, and they tend to lack champions and administrative support for a broader vision of how health IT fits into the overall picture of health care delivery. As a result, small providers can be at greater risk for not using health IT effectively and, more importantly, can fail to recognize and abate risks even after sentinel events.

Small practices and hospitals may often be more nimble than their larger counterparts in making changes to workflow processes and procedures, but they tend to lag in health IT implementation compared to large integrated delivery or hospital-based systems (see Box 4-3). Compared to their larger counterparts, small practices and hospitals generally have:

- Less administrative capacity or support to undertake the complex new process of health IT implementation and use (and no skills acquisition in this area during their medical training), especially with respect to workflow redesign to optimize the use of health IT (e.g., introduction of an e-prescribing system may require 26 separate mouse clicks to refill a prescription when only a few of those clicks may actually require a physician);
- Less redundancy in staff, which makes training more challenging and burdensome;
- Less capacity to support and train patients in use of new health IT products (e.g., these providers wind up becoming "help desks" for their patients using their IT such as secure email);
- Less access to technical support to keep their systems running reliably;
- Less ability to appreciate, purchase, and afford the amount of training and/or vendor support needed for an optimal implementation;
- Less capacity to monitor for and recognize new failure modes associated with implementation of health IT; and
- An absence of standard recommendations on a variety of key implementation issues such as what to do with paper, and whether to implement as a "big bang" or in phases.

---

[1] Ninety-three percent of all primary care physicians work in organizations of 10 physicians or fewer; of those, about half practice in organizations with 1 to 2 physicians (Bodenheimer and Pham, 2010).

BOX 4-3
A Small Provider's Experience with
Electronic Health Records (EHRs)

It was mostly on my initiative to implement an EHR. The process itself, which included five round-trip flights to Anchorage and 8 days off of work, was pricey and incredibly disappointing. Most EHRs were too expensive for small offices.

Of all my years in practice, the last year and a half has been my worst. Information is so poorly organized and difficult to access that I now have to remember that Ethel Smorley had an aorta that measured 4.2 cm on the ultrasound, which we did to follow up on her RUQ [right upper quadrant] abdominal pain. At the same time, I must remember that Thomas Richardson needs a RIBA [recombinant immunoblot assay], if and when the reagent becomes available, to sort out the meaning of his hepatitis C antibody.

For one patient I filed, a slightly elevated calcium with inappropriately normal PTH [parathyroid hormone] gets filed under "laboratory." I even took the time to label it "Ca + PTH-abnl-need short term f/u" so it stands out. Several months later when I look back at the lab-tab to review, that calcium and PTH are buried among all of the subsequent labs the patient has had and the date is off to the right of the "real estate" and without that all-important lateral scroll I can't tell if the lab was from a week ago or 4 years ago. To review the lab I have to click open one lab—wait one Mississippi, two Mississippi, three Mississippi—look, close, open the next— one Mississippi, two Mississippi, three Mississippi—look, close, open the next—one Mississippi, two Mississippi, three Mississippi—look, and close. It is easy to get lost.

For this patient I made an addendum to the chart noting the patient's complaint of depression and fatigue as well as the abnormal calcium and PTH and the need to follow up. But this addendum is in the virtual basement of the note and if you don't do a descending scroll down down down past the Assessment and Plan and the deceptive blank space beneath, the addendum isn't visible. You have to *know* it is there to find it, but if you *know* it is there you don't need to find it.

I copied a message from another patient's confidential and encrypted email and pasted it into his chart. I don't know how it happened but somehow it was also copied to a woman's chart. Now, according to my EHR, she is suffering from the same symptoms as the previous patient: scrotal pain, decreased urinary stream, and dysuria. It was tucked in the screen pocket out of sight and I immortalized it when I coded and closed the note. Now it lives there forever: A woman with scrotal pain.

If not for my familiarity with long-term patients, the luxury to schedule fewer patients in my day and survive the resultant financial hit, and the resilience of patients, I truly believe that bad outcomes could have happened. As I tell patients, I used to be a doctor but now I am a typist. I am fed up and frustrated and frightened of really missing something bad.

Personal communication, Elizabeth A. Kohnen, M.D., M.P.H., FACP, August 5, 2011.

Central to safe clinical implementation and use of health IT is adoption of redesigned workflows. With the adoption of health IT, each member of the office team or the staff within a small hospital setting needs to approach his job differently and use new tools, while also breaking up tasks and aligning them differently among team members. While this is true for all settings, the challenges of these processes are exacerbated in small practices and hospitals, which often have little to no experience in workflow redesign. New technologies simply inserted in old frameworks and workflows are likely to create new risks for patients.

Challenges also exist in both small practices and small hospitals with the integration of multiple health IT products from boutique niche software systems to legacy software systems. This is due in part to the proprietary nature of some products and the lack of adoption of data standards in other health IT products. The challenges to and costs of switching out vendors are prohibitive for small practices and hospitals, thus creating an obstacle for embracing new and improved technologies.

The great variability in implementation of health IT products in small provider settings is a major reason the literature is limited. Further research is needed to better understand the requirements specific to small practices and hospitals to enable safer deployment and use of health IT, such as the necessary resources and skills that facilitate the change-management process employed during health IT product implementation and adoption. In addition, small practices need self-assessment tools to evaluate the safety of their operational EHR systems.

Small Office Practices

Primary care physicians in small practices face particular challenges. They need to access, integrate, and interpret a large amount of data from multiple sources into a comprehensive picture of a patient. Much of these data are generated outside their offices (e.g., hospitals, specialists, laboratories, pathology laboratories) from information systems that are less likely to be integrated into their own record-keeping system.

In contrast, nonprimary care physicians may focus on more limited aspects of the patient's condition and are likely to generate much of the clinical data on which they need to act within their offices (e.g., a cardiac imaging machine produces structured data about relevant clinical issues such as left ventricular ejection fraction). Nonprimary care providers may also be more likely than primary care providers to have clinical support staff who assist with data entry, data aggregation, and data extraction in the routine course of patient care.

Small Hospitals

Small hospitals face many of the same challenges as small office practices. Typically there is limited expertise in health IT implementation, workflow redesign, and training, which is compounded by the fact that some small hospitals are struggling to implement the processes and technology needed to meet Health Information Technology for Economic and Clinical Health regulations. There can be large dependencies on vendor-supplied services and expertise, such as the following:

- Technology-related costs, in addition to the major investment needed for organizational and process change, challenge the small hospital already strapped with resource constraints necessary to maintain financial viability.
- Individuals with the required implementation process management expertise are either not present in sufficient numbers or are too immersed in other activities to devote the required time to a safe implementation.
- The small hospital has a huge challenge to assemble and organize the relatively large number of professionals required to ensure a successful implementation while at the same time ensuring that these participants' other responsibilities are met.
- Day-to-day participation by practicing physicians is especially problematic because small hospitals generally lack the complement of available clinical champions, physician administrators, hospital-based practitioners, intensivists, clinic directors, and training directors who often play critical roles in implementing clinical systems at larger institutions (Frisse and Metzer, 2005).

OPPORTUNITIES TO IMPROVE THE DESIGN AND DEVELOPMENT OF TECHNOLOGIES

Software development is an important determinant of patient safety in all types of health IT. Opportunities exist for vendors, aided by users, to improve safety in the different phases or activities of the software design and development life cycle. Although in theory these activities are identifiable, in practice the boundaries between them are not well defined and require varying levels of intensity to complete.

Health IT Vendor Design Activities

The key activities in the software life cycle are identifying requirements, software development and design, and testing (see Table 4-3).[2]

Software Requirements and Development Activities

Traditionally, the software development process begins with the explicit statement of what the software is intended to do and the circumstances under which such behavior is appropriate, otherwise known as the performance requirements. Clinicians communicate their needs in detailed statements based on evidence of safe practices whenever possible. Clinicians and software developers need to communicate safety needs and expectations for the clinical environment and the health IT product.

Traditional writing of requirements, although precise, can be a tedious task. When requirements become very complex, it is difficult to be confident that they actually describe what the users want. At times, a sequence of prototypes can be an alternative that allows users to see what a proposed version of the software would actually do. User input can provide for a more effective and accurate product. However, in a safety-critical area, even if the software task is defined by a sequence of prototypes, it will still be necessary to define the task sufficiently rigorously to permit adequate testing. The software functionality, whether developed from requirements or from experiments with prototypes, has to be understood as part of the process of delivering care and ought to reflect the desired changes to that process when it is revised and adapted in the light of operational experience.

Articulating requirements is often difficult. A critical path for identifying and validating requirements for software functionality includes assessment of current-state workflow, mapping the current state to the desired future state, and devising a plan to identify and address the gaps between the two. A process like this includes observation and documentation of the real-life workflow as well as interviews with the clinician. Validation that the software meets redesigned workflow needs is accomplished in multiple phases of testing to obtain iterative feedback from users, as discussed later in this chapter.

Many organizations purchasing health IT products define their requirements only once—immediately prior to purchasing the product off the shelf. Compared to organizations that can specify their requirements to their vendors, organizations purchasing products off the shelf face a somewhat

---

[2] Traditionally, these activities are called "phases" (e.g., requirements phase, design phase); this report adopts the "activities" terminology to emphasize the point that, although these activities are conceptually distinct, some of them may be occurring simultaneously from time to time.

TABLE 4-3
Health IT Vendor Design Activities

Activities/Phases	Features	Opportunities to Improve Safety
Requirements Activity	– Developers articulate what the software must do and the circumstances under which such behavior is appropriate – Developers articulate what the software must not do when safety is an issue – End users of the software must be intimately involved in all aspects of the requirements activity	– Clinicians communicate their needs – Clinicians identify data that must be captured or imported, with any requirements for conversion and validation such as full text entries – Prototype testing – Safety analyses
Software Development	– Involves actual programming or coding that reflects the software design – Software development is often undertaken iteratively with testing – Results from testing are used to inform another round of software development	– Iterative testing identifies unintended consequences for early revisions and informs the next round of development
Design of User Interface Activity	– Designers define the structure of the software – Software engineers decide on the appropriate technical approaches and solve problems conceptually	– Clinicians give feedback to designers about effectiveness or improvements needed for usability testing

TABLE 4-3 *Continued*

Activities/Phases	Features	Opportunities to Improve Safety

Testing Activity	– Examines the code that results from software development
	
	– Examines code functionality and the extent that the code complies with the requirements
	
	– Testing is often split into three separate subactivities:
	  • Unit testing, where individual software modules are tested
	  • Integration testing, where individual modules are assembled into an integrated whole and the whole assembly is tested
	  • Acceptance testing, where the entire assembly is tested to determine compliance with the requirements
		– Involving clinician superusers can reveal code functionality
		
		– Involving clinicians in the testing process provide an avenue for identification and correction of code defects and workflow risks
		
		– Dress rehearsals—real use by real users with actual data under realistic conditions—allow the clinicians opportunities to identify previously invisible flaws

NOTE: The design of user interfaces illustrates the concurrent nature of some of the activities of software development—users have an important stake in the design of user interfaces, and their needs must be expressed in the requirements activity.

different challenge—that of assessing whether an existing product is suitable for their organization.

Best practices for developing software emphasize systematicity and quality control. Software developers should identify and record significant risks of failure in development or in performance and articulate a plan to reduce them. They also need to have an explicit definition of the quality criteria for the software, to develop and follow version control procedures, and to track reported bugs and index them. Performing a complete safety analysis requires a comprehensive inventory of the possible clinical harms that might befall a patient and an understanding of how the health IT software might contribute to those harms.

Design of User Interface

Although definitive evidence is limited, the committee believes poor user-interface design is a threat to patient safety (Thimbleby, 2008; Thimbleby and Cairns, 2010). The user interface is one of the most important factors influencing the willingness of clinicians to interact with EHRs and to follow the intended use that is assumed to promote safe habits. The more functional the user interface, the more it enhances usability of the product. Inadequate user interfaces can lead to error and failure. The interface is intended to facilitate a desired clinical task; when the clinician cannot readily locate data or perceives the amount of time required to perform a function is too long, the user interface needs to be evaluated. Poor interface design that detracts from clinician efficiency and affinity for the system will likely lead to under-use or misuse of the system (Franzke, 1995).

The goals of user-centered design are to create an efficient, effective, and satisfying interaction with the user. The interface design starts with an understanding of human behaviors and familiar work patterns. Human nature is such that busy clinicians will trade thoroughness for efficiency, or they will modify their behavior to achieve efficiency. Shneiderman has identified eight heuristically and experientially derived "golden rules" for interface design that, if followed, support the principles of EHR usability (Shneiderman et al., 2009), including consistency for similar tasks; universal applicability for a wide range of expertise; feedback for every user action; communicating closure of an action sequence; design to prevent errors; allowing easy reversal of actions; avoiding complex data entry and retrieval sequences; and reducing memory load (see Table 4-1). Although it is important to develop and follow principles for safe design interfaces, it is equally important that designers do not follow a formulaic checklist. Instead, designers need to continually interact with users to discover and address the safety issues unique to each clinical environment. Formal usability testing during development is essential.

In Vivo Testing: Uncovering Use Error Versus User Error

Often, miscommunications between developers and users leave critical ambiguities that can only be discovered through testing. Therefore, it is critical to test health IT during *all stages* of development to determine whether user requirements have been translated into software that actually does what the user wants. An important source of information for obtaining information about meeting clinician needs is operational prototype testing. The first versions of software rarely meet clinician needs fully, and observing how a clinician uses a software prototype will yield a great deal of information about what the clinician actually does and does not find useful and appropriate. Such observations are fed back to software developers, who then revise the software so that its performance better reflects user needs and safe practices as expressed in an operational context.

However, testing cannot be oriented solely to determining if software does what it is supposed to do when users follow all of the proper steps. Because users do make mistakes, a significant portion of testing must be devoted to seeing if the software responds properly when the user does something unexpected. For example, the user may enter data in an unexpected format. Testing is also a longer-term process where the experiences of users based on reported events and workarounds is considered as part of a postmarketing program designed to improve the design of software. To maximize the user–designer feedback loop, EHR products might include a "report here now" button on each screen wherein the user can indicate that a display was confusing, a workflow was cumbersome, or some other way that the design did not support optimal clinical care.

Software Implementation and Postdeployment Activities

Portions of the software life cycle led by vendors in partnership with users influence safer use of health IT such as training prior to implementation, addressing problems that appear during testing and implementation of software, and planning for the ongoing maintenance and upgrade activities that directly impact users. These activities occur not only as part of software development but also during implementation and subsequent phases of use in an organization (see Table 4-4).

Software Implementation Activity

After the technology package is deemed ready for delivery to the user, it is transmitted to the user's organization for initial use. Prior to using health IT products in the care of patients, extensive training must be done for the specific product and the specific organizational setting. It is customary for organizations to set expectations for training that require documentation of learning modules and demonstrated competency. Resources to support initial and ongoing training are essential components of planned implementation activities. The period of initial use in an operational environment is fraught with patient safety risks, because it is during this period that many problems are most likely to appear. Some of these problems will result from users who have not received adequate training—this will be true even if the technology is designed to require minimal training. Other problems will result from operating the technology with the health of real patients at stake rather than in an artificial environment that is well controlled and does not reflect an actual health care setting.

TABLE 4-4
Health IT Vendor Implementation and Postdeployment Activities

Activities/Phases	Features	Opportunities to Improve Safety
Software Implementation Activity	– Installing the software in the users' organization – Users are trained to use the software	– Initial planning involves end users prior to deployment – Training is provider- or user-specific to achieve desired learning

Maintenance Activity	– Fixing problems that appear after deployment, including errors that may have occurred during
	  • Software implementation (i.e., programming errors)
	  • Requirements (i.e., incorrect elicitation of performance requirements from users)
	  • Design (e.g., a dysfunctional architecture)
		– Mechanism for rapid identification of needed maintenance will avoid perpetuating flaws
		– Performing episodic maintenance maintains trust by users
		– Planned maintenance is best practice

Upgrade Activity	Modifying the software to meet new requirements that may emerge over time, such as enabling the software to work with new hardware	– Planning for upgrades with adequate backup systems is a requirement – Planned safety testing of operational system on routine ongoing basis

NOTE: Traditionally, these activities are called "phases" (e.g., requirements phase, design phase); this report adopts the "activities" terminology to emphasize the point that, although these activities are conceptually distinct, some of them may be occurring simultaneously from time to time.

An organization typically selects one of two approaches to implementing the technology: either a big bang strategy (i.e., the technology is implemented for use throughout the entire organization at the same time or nearly so) or an incremental approach (i.e., the technology is first deployed for use on a small scale within the organization and then, as operating experience is acquired, it is deployed to other parts of the organization in a gradual, staged manner).

Experience with the implementation of large-scale technology applications suggests that, over time, success is possible with either approach. Nevertheless, a health care organization should plan on the simultaneous operation of both the new and old technologies (even if the old technology is paper based) for some transitional period, so that failures in the new technology do not cripple the organization. Backup and contingency plans are necessary to help anticipate and protect against a wide range of failures and problems with the newly implemented technology and are an essential part of implementation planning.

Maintenance and Upgrade Activities

Maintenance and upgrade refer to activities carried out after software is initially deployed to keep it operational, to support ongoing use, or to add new functionality to the software. Because upgrading a software package involves many of the same considerations as maintenance, the discussion that follows will speak simply of "maintenance" with the understanding that the term also includes upgrades. During maintenance, health IT products are continuously subject to a variety of activities and interventions by vendors intended to correct defects, introduce new features, optimize performance, or adapt to changing user environment or technologies (Canfora et al., 2010).

Maintenance activities paradoxically can make products increasingly defect-laden and more difficult to understand and maintain in the future (Parnas, 1994). Maintenance activities inadvertently tend to degrade software system structure, increase source code complexity, and produce a net negative effect on system design for a variety of reasons, such as production pressures, limited resource allocation, and the lack of a disciplined process. Maintenance also increases the complexity of health IT, increasing the likelihood for error.

End users and purchasers of health IT are not always aware of the specific risks associated with the maintenance phase. Installation of a patch (code upgrade) can disrupt existing functionality by introducing previously absent dependencies, and functionality can be lost by installing a patch. Maintenance work often requires taking software offline for a number of hours, and requires advance planning and notification of users to minimize disruptions in care. Maintenance also requires that actively engaged users be involved in the testing process prior to the implementation of a patch or upgrade into the production environment.

OPPORTUNITIES TO IMPROVE SAFETY IN THE USE OF HEALTH IT

Safer use is intimately linked to safer design. For example, safer use of an EHR evolves from effective planning and deployment with testing and management of human–computer interface issues, to optimization of tools and processes to improve the application of the system. Users receive education and skill development to learn the utility of the system and accept responsibility to report conditions that could detract from or enhance EHR functionality. Observation, measurement, and synthesis of lessons learned about the impact of EHRs on desired work patterns and outputs will help address deficiencies in the design, usability, and clinical behavior related to EHR products. Ensuring safer use relies upon evaluation of workload impact—ergonomic, cognitive, and data comprehension—and its effect on each clinician and the care team. There is a need for metrics to describe accurately user interactions with EHRs and other health IT devices that enable care (Armijo et al., 2009). For users, the opportunities to improve safety of health IT can be divided into the following phases: acquisition, clinical implementation (which includes planning and goal setting, deployment, stabilization, optimization, and transformation), and maintenance activities (see Table 4-5). These stages create a continuous cycle that can be applied throughout the life cycle of health IT. The safety of health IT is contingent on each of these stages. An ongoing commitment to implementation is needed to realize safer, more effective care. It is an iterative process that requires ongoing learning and improvement based on the experience of users.

Acquisition

The first activity for users is the decision to move from an existing environment or status quo to one that better serves the business needs and/or functionalities of the organization or practice. Delineation of business needs and drivers is the foundation of the IT strategy that propels the decision to acquire a system and initiates the acquisition process. Acquiring health IT requires a decision and commitment to change workflows within the organization. Designing new and acceptable workflows, training staff, and dealing with consequential changes will be major drivers of cost and potential risk. Implementing a new health IT product is not an IT project, it is a quality improvement and business change project facilitated by IT.

A needs assessment can help evaluate the current status and the future needs in relation to the health IT solutions targeted to close gaps in clinical, operational, and financial goals. After a need is identified, timelines for acquiring and implementing ought to be developed and an imperative for change be created. Change management is complex and requires organizations to be aware of the potential downstream misalignments between the perceived functionality of health IT and the needs of the organization.

Acquisition requires a deliberative process to select and attain a system that will connect data from clinical and other related IT and support an organization's clinical and administrative workflows. The organization wants to ensure an effective, safe implementation and not favor speed over quality; the number of systems being integrated may also affect the depth and volume of implementation support required. Similarly, the cost of a health

TABLE 4-5
Health IT User Activities

Activities/Phases	Features	Opportunities to Improve Safety
Acquisition	– Selecting and attaining a system that will connect data from clinical and other related IT and support an organization's clinical and administrative workflows	– Perform self-assessments and strategic planning before the decision to purchase health IT – Ensure that the resources needed to support adoption and implementation of health IT products are available

Clinical Implementation	– Planning and goal setting
	  • Assessing needs
	  • Selecting systems based on functionality
	  • Testing quality before go-live
	– Deployment
	  • Training and demonstrating competence of users
	  • Converting data conversions prior to go-live
	  • Minimizing mix of electronic and paper functions
	  • Planning orderly implementation
	– Stabilization
	  • Evaluating human-computer interactions for effective design and interface
	  • Correcting functions that disrupt workflow
	  • Minimizing downtime
	  • Planning maintenance
	– Optimization
	  • Engaging clinical decision support
	  • Retraining for proper and best use
	  • Readdressing changes needed for workflow improvements
	– Transformation
	  • Measuring improved clinical and efficiency outcomes
		– Analyze existing workflow, envision the optimal workflow, and select the automated system that achieves the optimal automated workflow
		– Establish mechanisms and metrics to identify, escalate, and remediate patient safety issues
		– Testing locally to verify safety, interoperability, security, and effectiveness
		– Monitor and measure the dependability, reliability, and security of the installed system
		– Take steps to resolve any potential hazards
		– Learn and improve patient safety by utilizing data generated by the health IT system

continued

TABLE 4-5 *Continued*

Activities/Phases	Features	Opportunities to Improve Safety
Maintenance Activities	– Activities are carried out to keep a system operational and to support ongoing use	– Schedule any needed downtown and upgrades in advance to minimize disruptions in workflow
		– Establish workflow procedures for scheduled and/or unexpected downtime

IT product is often a major driver in the decision-making process, but cost has to be balanced with quality of the product. Maintenance costs also need to be recognized. Unconstrained growth of requirements can result in changing project goals that can lead to frustration and schedule overruns.

Organizations should perform self-assessments and strategic planning before the decision to purchase health IT. Organizations need to consider their innovation temperance, or their tolerance for risk, as well as the stability of the current process. Organizational infrastructure also needs to be considered to ensure that the resources needed to support adoption and implementation of health IT products are available. Not only are the personnel resources and monetary resources important but also the technical resources needed to adopt the proposed technology, such as the ability to test the product and ensure functionality including interoperability with secure exchange of data. The characteristics of having a culture of safety, being a learning organization, having strong staff morale, and having adequate resources are critical to the successful adoption of health IT. These are especially important for smaller organizations with fewer resources to consider in the adoption and decision-making processes. Much of the responsibility for these characteristics occurs at the senior leadership level, but driving change requires both administrative and clinical staff taking on delineated roles.

These antecedents to acquisition will help an organization prepare for both acquisition and implementation of health IT and optimize outcomes in subsequent phases of the implementation life cycle. Unfortunately, sometimes the due process of strategic planning is in place, but the evaluative decision-making model is inadequate. For example, everyone's opinions and feedback are acquired by the organization leaders, but, in the final decision, critical information from the clinicians may be weighted the least (Keselman et al., 2004).

Some of the generalizable traits organizations must demonstrate for achieving safer patient care have applicability to the use of health IT. Gleaned from sociotechnical industries such as aviation, nuclear power, chemical, road transportation, and health care, there are five systemic needs health care providers must satisfy to maximize safe performance, which are the needs to:

- Limit the discretion of workers,
- Reduce worker autonomy,
- Transition from a craftsmanship mindset to that of equivalent actors,
- Develop system-level (senior leadership) arbitration to optimize safety strategies, and
- Strive for simplification (Amalberti et al., 2005).

At times, these restraining forces are at odds with traditional values promoting autonomy, creativity, academic expression, safety, and exercising professional judgment. They do, however, demand careful consideration to ensure the very individuals entrusted to provide safe care are not contributing barriers to safe care delivery.

An organization's readiness to adopt health IT can impact the safety, suitability, and performance of the technology. Managing end-user expectations from the beginning will also help aid implementation. Clinicians expect technology to be perfect and deliver efficient and effective information just in time, every time, with little effort. Whereas most systems are able to perform at these levels, there will be times, such as initial implementation or unanticipated downtimes, that will challenge user patience. These factors need to be considered before implementation both to reduce burdens to the organization and to protect the organization from harming patients in the later phases.

Clinical Implementation

Successful deployment of a health IT product and its effective use are intended to achieve seamless internal information flow as well as to enhance performance in safety, quality, service, and cost. Safe implementation of health IT is a complex, dynamic process that requires continual feedback to vendors and investment by health care organizations. Merely installing health information technologies in health care organizations will not result in improvements in care.

Because each health care organization is different, each organization has different needs and makes choices resulting in varied, customized implementation. Poor implementation can result in the development of processes different from the intended use of a system, otherwise known as use error.

As shown in Figure 4-2, implementation includes the stages of planning and goal setting, deployment, stabilization, optimization, and transformation.

Planning and Goal Setting

In planning and goal setting, organizations target improvements in quality, safety, and efficiency when automating processes. For example, automating orders or medication administration targets improvements of systems composed of nonlinear, complex workflows. The first step is similar to the acquisition phase—determining the organization's needs and identifying the resources needed to achieve those needs. In aligning technological and organizational change, there needs to be effective management of both technological and organizational change (Majchrzak and Meshkati, 2001). The organization needs to analyze existing workflow, envision the optimal workflow, and select the automated system that achieves the optimal automated workflow. This may involve customization of the purchased system. If workflow analysis and redesign are not completed before implementation, it is possible automation will create unanticipated safety risks. For example, the introduction of a new lab system may require new work and the right person to take on that new work may not have been correctly selected, resulting in the new work falling to the physician or others at the cost of other clinical activities.

Users need to be actively involved in the planning and goal-setting stage. Mechanisms to identify, escalate, and remediate patient safety issues need to be in place as the organization proceeds to the deployment stage. Metrics to be considered at this stage include ensuring that organization leaders have identified objectives, teams, and resources committed to the implementation.

Deployment

When organizations deploy a selected health IT, they make assumptions that vendors have made safety a primary goal in specification and design, that their products support high-reliability processes, and health IT standards (e.g., content, vocabulary, transport) have evolved to address safety, safe use, and value (McDonnell et al., 2010). At the same time, strategies are needed to address potential patient-safety events that can arise from decisions such as whether the organization should take a big bang or sequential approach and how to manage partial paper and electronic systems that can create opportunities for missing data and communication lapses.

Collaboration between user organizations and vendors to improve patient safety is critical and requires a specific and immediate information loop between the parties, allowing detailed information to be exchanged to

I: Planning/Goal Setting	II: Deployment	III: Stabilization	IV: Optimization	V: Transformation
- What are we hoping to achieve? - What are our criteria for success? - What training is valuable and needed? - What are the roles for champions and governance?	- Is it installed? - How many users are up? - Is it running?	- Is it reliable? - Are users proficient enough?	- Is the "build" optimal? - Have we improved workflows? - Are we improving quality, service, and cost of care?	- Are we creating a new value proposition for patients? - Are we supporting an ongoing learning health care organization?

Factors That Enhance or Detract from Patient Safety

- Are users actively involved in the acquisition and design of the system?
- What are the mechanisms to identify, escalate, and remediate patient safety issues and errors as deployment proceeds?
- How does patient safety remain a major organizational and provider priority?
- Do the design principles increase safety or generate measures that verify usable design?
- Are safety enhancements standardized across all users (response, formats, data presentation, colors, etc.)?
- What systems (past and present) will interface with EHRs?
- Does the culture encourage users' willingness to report safety concerns?

- Is big bang or sequential safer?
- How to best retrofit paper into electronic?
- "Old data" conversion
- Training strategies: what frequency and targeted content?
- What quality testing is sufficient for interfaces? And go-lives?
- Who is clinically accountable to follow up on data?
  - Who fixes bad data?
  - Who fixes new "bad" habits (i.e., potentially harmful shortcuts and egregious behavior)?
- How will the organization track and address new work created by the EHR (i.e., unintended consequences of work flow changes)?

- How are "downtimes" managed?
- When do downtimes become hazardous?
- When can a user be deemed proficient enough to ensure patient safety?
- Are human-computer interactions being managed to avoid hazards and create safe use?
  - fatigue, impatience, stress, switching off alerts
  - communication hazards
  - difficult user interface
  - "paste forward" and other user-developed shortcuts
- Is system dependable, available, reliable, and secure?
- When a user-computer interaction leads to a potential hazard, how will the organization resolve the underlying problem rather than blame the user?

- What clinical decision support is important to have?
- What other mechanisms improve patient safety now that EHR is installed?
- What principles and policies are in place for sound stewardship of secondary data use?
- Is there an iterative review of workflow process for the task distribution to the care team as a result of the technology deployment?

- How do we learn about errors, hazards that occur in the organization?
  - ...outside the organization with the same vendor product?
  - ...and how do we remediate as quickly as possible?
- How do we test operational system after annual upgrades or crashes to ensure that it is still performing safely?

FIGURE 4-2
Implementation life cycle.

SOURCE: Adapted from Kaiser Permanente experience.

quickly address safety issues or potential safety issues. Attention to collateral impact in a multivendor environment is also necessary to identify any other corrective actions. For example, in the event a safety incident occurs, rapid notification of health IT stakeholders should be accompanied by rapid correction of system-safety flaws, including vendor notification and collaboration to change software, process, or policy as indicated. Most mechanisms impose a large burden on users to specify what was happening when a problem occurred (e.g., a system error, an instance of inconvenient use, an instance of avoidable provider error). The organization should consider developing mechanisms for providing feedback from users to vendors in an easy-to-use way, such as a "report problem here" button on every screen.

Local testing is needed to verify safety, interoperability, security, and effectiveness, particularly at interfaces with other software systems during the go-live event. Policies to define data stewardship need to address accountability for following up on data when there is more than one recipient, development of processes for correcting incorrect data, and ways to identify and avoid potentially harmful shortcuts or behaviors that result in unintended use of the system. Ongoing monitoring to assure secure exchange of data as well as adherence to predetermined security performance expectations is essential; users must have confidence that data are secure at all times. General metrics for evaluating deployment include failure rates, quality assurance rates for each interface, percentage of users trained, and checklists of essential functions.

Clinicians using multiple EHRs also experience challenges of retaining information about how to use different EHR systems. This affects professionals in training as well as those on staff who care for patients in multiple settings or organizations.

Stabilization

Following deployment, health IT enters a stage of stabilization. During stabilization, potentially hazardous human–computer interactions such as alert fatigue, communication hazards, and workarounds such as "paste forward" must be managed. During this stage, the organization ought to be monitoring the dependability, reliability, and security of the installed system and taking steps to resolve any potential hazards. More specific measures of these system characteristics will guide actions for clinician retraining, software modification, and the need for additional guidance and policies. As with the maintenance activity in the design and development of technology, stabilization also provides time to evaluate how downtime is managed. Organizations can measure the stability of a system by assessing user proficiency (e.g., reduction in helpdesk calls, higher percentage of e-prescriptions), the percentage of time the system is available, and trends in identified errors for a given timeframe.

Optimization

In the optimization stage, the organization analyzes how well it is using the functions such as decision support and safety effects of computerized provider order entry (CPOE) and other functions. Revisiting revised workflows to measure achievement of intended changes can reveal improvements or degradation in quality and service. Assessing task distribution to the care team can help evaluate the impact of the health IT. Further evaluation is important to assess changes in quality measures over time as well as whether the health IT is being used in a meaningful manner. One example of measuring optimization is by tracking quality over time and the level of an organization's reliance on paper. Self-assessment tools are an important adjunct approach to assessing aspects of EHR use such as clinical decision support performance (Metzger et al., 2010). A sample set of concepts for metrics to track a successful implementation across the life cycle of an EHR appears in Table 4-6.

Transformation: The Learning Health System

Transformation is the future state of an organization that has extracted learning from the system itself and from application of knowledge. It can be evaluated by identifying changes in practice derived from aggregate data analysis and application of new knowledge that result in improved outcomes. Proactive monitoring for new failure modes created by the implementation and use of health IT is going to be necessary. Proactive monitoring can also help define how such failures occur, and the contributing forces. In the small practice and hospital setting this is particularly challenging because there is limited to no experience in these methods or approaches.

A learning health care organization creates a new value proposition by improving quality and value of care. Ultimately the transformation achieved through optimal use of health IT will improve outcomes over time and achieve a safer system. Continuous evaluation and improvement occurs over the dynamic and iterative life cycle of health IT products (Walker et al., 2008).

Maintenance Activities

Maintenance begins after implementation when activities are carried out to keep a system operational and to support ongoing use. It is a period

TABLE 4-6
Measure Concepts for Successful Implementation

I Planning and Goal Setting	II Deployment	III Stabilization	IV Optimization	V Transformation
- IT, medical, and operations leaders identified and in agreement on objectives - Teams identified - Money and resources made available	- System up - Percentage of users trained - Percentage of users logged in - Number and nature of errors identified in the field per week - Quality assurance stats for each interface - Quality assurance user acceptance testing stats for system - "Shakedown cruise" stats—review of functionality in initial period post go-live	- Percentage of time system is available - User proficiency measures - Trend of errors identified in the field per week - Alert overrides - Event reports	- Ongoing health IT patient safety with analysis of reporting and remediation of safety issue - Tracking of quality measures over time - Quality improvement (QI) projects and results - System passes ongoing safety tests after all upgrades, crashed or new application implementations	- Show improved outcomes over time - Health care is safer based on identified measures - Care processes redesigned - Continuous improvement of new steady state

when there is shared responsibility between the vendor and the organization. The cost and effort needed to maintain an IT system is influenced by the underlying complexity of the system and design choices made by both vendors and users. A relationship exists between the complexity of the system and the error-proneness of a system immediately after installation. Complexity also increases the overall lifetime effort and cost associated with maintenance activities.

Contingency planning for downtime procedures and data loss is necessary to address both short- and long-term occurrences. Scheduled downtime for maintenance and upgrades typically occurs at the organization's discretion to minimize work disruption. Downtime procedures for planned outages as well as emergency procedures are necessary to protect security and are to include measures to prevent data loss; these measures will differ based on the type of EHR architecture. Planning for obsolescence and eventual system replacement also requires a contingency plan that includes safeguarding of data (American Academy of Family Physicians, 2011). Any disruption, no matter how small, can present safety risks resulting from unfamiliarity with manual backup systems, delays in care, and data loss. Power interruptions and other unexpected events can result in unavoidable downtime. Procedures should address immediate communication and deployment of contingency plans as well as reentry to normal functioning and subsequent recovery actions. Advance planning, education, training, and practice for downtime can aid in successful performance during planned or unplanned outages.

MINIMIZING RISKS OF HEALTH IT TO PROMOTE SAFER CARE

Although not everything is known about the risks of health IT, there is some evidence to suggest there will be failures, design flaws, and user behaviors that thwart safe performance and application of these systems. To better understand these failures, more research, training, and education will be needed. Specifically, measures of safe practices need to be developed to assess health IT safety. Vendors, health care providers, and organizations could benefit from following a proven set of general safe practices representing the best evidence about design, implementation strategies, usability features, and human-computer interactions for optimizing safe use. Vendors take primary responsibility for the design and development of technologies with iterative feedback from users. Users assume responsibility for safe implementation and work with vendors through the health IT life cycle. The mutual exchange of ideas and feedback regarding any actual or potential failures or unintended consequences can also inform safer design and use of health IT products.

Because of the variations in health IT products and their implementation, a set of development requirements that stipulates consistent criteria known to produce safer design and user interactions would be beneficial. Consistent testing procedures could then be applied to ensure the safety of health IT products. Inclusion of appropriate requirements and iterative testing can contribute to effective practices for safe design and implementation.

With growing experience of health IT and EHR deployment, gleaning best practices for implementation from case reports and reviews is possible. The importance of testing for safe designs, functioning, and usability to reduce deployment errors can enhance safety in user adoption. Continual testing and retesting, for any change such as when upgrades are installed, will be needed. As high-prevalence and high-impact EHR-related patient safety risks are identified, these should be incorporated into pre- and postdeployment testing. Feedback from testing as well as learning from event reports and detecting workarounds is also important as part of the iterative process of continually improving health IT.

The partnership to design, develop, implement, and optimize systems extends beyond a single vendor and single organization. Many public- and private-sector groups have a stake in the safety of health IT to ensure the very systems intended to help improve quality of care are performing without creating risk of harm. Indeed such a public–private partnership already exists in this area through the National Quality Forum's safe practices, one of which is focused on CPOE and includes in its standard the routine use of a postdeployment test of the safety of operational CPOE systems in hospitals (Classen et al., 2010). Ensuring this outcome will entail additional requirements for public and private agencies, vendors, and users across the health IT life cycle.

Current government programs, such as EHR product certification, can also be a path toward more effective usability and safer use of health IT products. Together, product developers, certification groups, and the Office of the National Coordinator for Health IT (ONC) can expand product requirements that address safer deployment with strategies to mitigate anticipated risks and address those that develop unexpectedly. Accrediting agencies can reinforce relevant standards and criteria for safer health IT by including review criteria for areas such as training, standardized testing procedures, maintenance, and safety issue reporting and remediation internally and with vendors. Vigilance before, during, and after the selection and implementation of health IT is a shared responsibility.

Data from EHRs also can be used to evaluate the impact of health IT on patient safety. Methods for collecting and evaluating these data are needed.

Recommendation 1: The Secretary of Health and Human Services (HHS) should publish an action and surveillance plan within 12 months that includes a schedule for working with the private sector to assess

the impact of health IT on patient safety and minimizing the risk of its implementation and use. The plan should specify:

a. The Agency for Healthcare Research and Quality (AHRQ) and the National Library of Medicine (NLM) should expand their funding of research, training, and education of safe practices as appropriate, including measures specifically related to the design, implementation, usability, and safe use of health IT by all users, including patients.

b. The ONC should expand its funding of processes that promote safety that should be followed in the development of health IT products, including standardized testing procedures to be used by manufacturers and health care organizations to assess the safety of health IT products.

c. The ONC and AHRQ should work with health IT vendors and health care organizations to promote postdeployment safety testing of EHRs for high-prevalence, high-impact EHR-related patient safety risks.

d. Health care accrediting organizations should adopt criteria relating to EHR safety.

e. AHRQ should fund the development of new methods for measuring the impact of health IT on safety using data from EHRs.

CONCLUSION

Building health IT for safer use by health professionals is indeed a shared responsibility. Vendors, care providers, provider organizations and their health IT departments, and public and private agencies focused on quality of care are all partners in building a safer system in which health IT is used. The recommendations outlined in this chapter seek to align this shared responsibility and to provide structured guidance to further support safer care enabled by health IT. The committee acknowledges that health IT is an evolving domain and, as such, guidance, structure, and processes will need to evolve as well.

REFERENCES

Amalberti, R., Y. Auroy, D. Berwick, and P. Barach. 2005. Five system barriers to achieving ultrasafe health care. *Annals of Internal Medicine* 142(9):756-764.

American Academy of Family Physicians. 2011. *Develop a contingency plan for down time and data loss.* http://www.centerforhit.org/online/chit/home/cme-learn/tutorials/networking/network201/contingency.printerview.html (accessed June 28, 2011).

Armijo, D., C. McDonnell, and K. Werner. 2009. *Electronic health record usability: Interface design considerations.* Rockville, MD: Agency for Healthcare Research and Quality.

Berwick, D. 2003. Disseminating innovations in health care. *Journal of the American Medical Association* 289(15):1969-1975.

Bodenheimer, T., and H. H. Pham. 2010. Primary care: Current problems and proposed solutions. *Health Affairs* 29(5):799-805.

Canfora, G., L. Cerulo, M. Di Penta, and F. Pacilio. 2010. *An exploratory study of factors influencing change entropy.* Paper presented at 2010 IEEE 18th International Conference on Program Comprehension (ICPC), June 30 to July 2, 2010.

Card, S., T. Moran, and A. Newell. 1983. *The psychology of human–computer interaction.* Hillsdale, NJ: Lawrence Erlbaum.

Classen, D. C., D. W. Bates, and C. R. Denham. 2010. Meaningful use of computerized prescriber order entry. *Journal of Patient Safety* 6(1):15-23.

Franzke, M. 1995. *Turning research into practice: Characteristics of display-based interaction.* Paper presented at the SIGCHI Conference on Human Factors in Computing Systems, Denver, CO, May 7, 1995.

Frisse, M. E., and J. Metzer. 2005. Information technology in the rural setting: Challenges and more challenges. *Journal of the American Medical Informatics Association* 12(1):99-100.

Hoekstra, M., M. Vogelzang, E. Verbitskiy, and M. W. N. Nijsten. 2009. Health technology assessment review: Computerized glucose regulation in the intensive care unit—how to create artificial control. *Critical Care* 13(5):223.

John, B., K. Prevas, D. Salvucci, and K. Koedinger. 2004. *Predictive human performance modeling made easy.* Paper presented at the Conference on Human Factors in Computing Systems, Vienna, Austria, April 24 to 29, 2004.

Kaelber, D. C., A. K. Jha, D. Johnston, B. Middleton, and D. W. Bates. 2008. A research agenda for personal health records (PHRs). *Journal of the American Medical Informatics Association* 15(6):729-736.

Keselman, A., X. Tang, V. L. Patel, T. R. Johnson, and J. Zhang. 2004. Institutional decision-making for medical device purchasing: Evaluating patient safety. *Medinfo* 11:1357-1361.

Kieras, D. (unpublished). *Using the keystroke-level model to estimate execution times.*

Koppel, R., T. Wetterneck, J. L. Telles, and B. T. Karsh. 2008. Workarounds to barcode medication administration systems: Their occurrences, causes, and threats to patient safety. *Journal of the American Medical Informatics Association* 15(4):408-423.

Majchrzak, A. and N. Meshkati. 2001. Aligning technological and organizational change when implementing new technology. In *The handbook of industrial engineering,* 3rd ed, edited by G. Salvendy. New York: Wiley. Pp. 948-974.

McDonnell, C., K. Werner, and L. Wendel. 2010. *Electronic health record usability: Vendor practices and perspectives.* Rockville, MD: Agency for Healthcare Research and Quality.

Metzger, J., E. Welebob, D. W. Bates, S. Lipsitz, and D. C. Classen. 2010. Mixed results in the safety performance of computerized physician order entry. *Health Affairs* 29(4):655-663.

Neilson, J. 1994. *Usability engineering.* San Diego, CA: Academic Press.

NIST (National Institute of Standards and Technology). 2010a. *Customized common industry format template for electronic health record usability testing.* Gaithersburg, MD: NIST.

NIST. 2010b. *NIST guide to the processes approach for improving the usability of electronic health records.* Gaithersburg, MD: NIST.

NIST. 2011. *Technical evaluation, testing and validation of the usability of electronic health records.* Gaithersburg, MD: NIST.

NRC (National Research Council). 2009. *Compuational technology for effective health care: Immediate steps and strategic directions.* Washington, DC: The National Academies Press.

Parnas, D. L. 1994. *Software aging.* Paper presented at the 16th International Conference on Software Engineering, Sorrento, Italy, May 16 to 21, 1994.

Shneiderman, B., C. Plaisant, M. Cohen, and S. Jacobs. 2009. *Designing the user interface: Strategies for effective human-computer interaction.* Boston: Addison-Wesley.

Thimbleby, H. 2008. Ignorance of interaction programming is killing people. *Interactions* 15(5):52-57.

Thimbleby, H., and P. Cairns. 2010. Reducing number entry errors: Solving a widespread, serious problem. *Journal of The Royal Society Interface* 7(51):1429-1439.

Walker, J. M., P. Carayon, N. Leveson, R. A. Paulus, J. Tooker, H. Chin, A. Bothe, Jr., and W. F. Stewart. 2008. EHR safety: The way forward to safe and effective systems. *Journal of the American Medical Informatics Association* 15(3):272-277.

Zhang, J., and M. Walji. 2011. TURF: Toward a unified framework of EHR usability. *Journal of Biomedical Informatics* 44(6):1056-1067.

Zhang, J., T. R. Johnson, V. L. Patel, D. L. Paige, and T. Kubose. 2003. Using usability heuristics to evaluate patient safety of medical devices. *Journal of Biomedical Informatics* 36(1-2):23-30.

5

Patients' and Families' Use of Health IT: Concerns About Safety

While much of the focus of this report is on health IT products that are intended to support clinicians and health care delivery organizations, health IT products are also being developed to engage and support patients in health-related decision making and management of their own personal health information. This chapter discusses a few of these tools, which are often seen as supporting patient engagement and the relationship, if any, between use of these tools and patient safety.

PATIENT-CENTERED CARE AND THE ROLE OF HEALTH IT

Patient-centered care, and patient and family engagement in health care, has been a growing priority in national health policy discussions. The Institute of Medicine (IOM) identified patient-centeredness as one of the six aims of quality health care (IOM, 2001). Federal and private-sector agents have echoed this patient-centered focus in several recent policy and position statements. The National Quality Forum's National Priorities Partnership, for example, has called for care that is both patient-centered and engages patients and their families (NQF, 2011), and the Department of Health and Human Services' National Quality Strategy declared as a priority "that each person and family is engaged as partners in their care" (HHS, 2011). More recently the discussion also has focused on the role that information technology can play in achieving some patient-engagement goals. In its 2010 report, the President's Council of Advisors on Science and Technology asserted that health information technology "can help patients become more involved in their own care, which is especially important in managing chronic conditions" (PCAST, 2010). Consistent with this, the Office of the National Coordinator for Health Information Technology (ONC) included a goal of "empower[ing] individuals with health IT to improve their health and the health care system" in its draft federal health IT strategic plan (ONC, 2011) and has included this goal in the criteria for its meaningful use program.

Over time, discussions of patient or family engagement in health care have tended to revolve around three topics:

1. Patients' access to their own personal health data in electronic formats (personal health information management);
2. Patients' access to evidence-based information about their medical conditions, treatment options, and health-promoting activities and behaviors (more than 80 percent of Internet users in the United States search for health information online (Pew Research Center, 2011); and
3. Effective communication between a patient (and family or care-giver) and health care providers and the health care delivery system so as to improve safety and quality.

Such discussions center on the belief that patients who have the tools to manage their own health care data, who have ready access to reliable health-related information, and/or who can communicate more effectively with health professionals will be capable of making more informed decisions and will experience better outcomes. Recent trends with personal health records (PHRs) indicate that patient engagement tools may have a role in allowing patients and their families to become more involved in their care. Therefore, the impact of the growing use of patient engagement tools on patient safety should be considered.

GROWTH OF CONSUMER HEALTH IT

There has been rapid growth of consumer health IT in recent years designed for the purpose of enabling patients and their families to become truly engaged consumers of health care (Poon et al., 2007). Tools such as PHRs can help patients feel more knowledgeable about their conditions, offer shared decision making, and can lead to fewer gaps in care (California HealthCare Foundation, 2010; Detmer et al., 2008; Zhou et al., 2010). For example, one study found that patients had eight times more adverse events than noted in their medical records when asked directly if they had experienced a problem with a drug (Gandhi et al., 2003). Importantly, PHRs can also be used to improve communications between patients and health professionals.

It is reasonable to assume that, over time, patient interest in health IT resources will increase, especially given the broad appeal of general Internet use, including social networking and other consumer-oriented web services. Among American health care consumers, considerable interest exists in Internet access to personal health information stored on electronic health records (EHRs). Across several surveys, 76 to 86 percent of respondents expressed interest in having access to their health information over the Internet (Fricton and Davies, 2008; Patel et al., 2010; Wen et al., 2010); however, at that time, 1 in 11 had experience doing so (Wen et al., 2010). It has been found that people pay more attention to and become more engaged in their health and medical care when they have easy online access to their health information (Skorve, 2010).

In addition, patient "engagement" and "centeredness" have become ubiquitous goals and objectives of many policies and programs promoted by health reform. For many engaged in realizing these goals, widespread adoption and use of health IT by the public is a necessary, if not sufficient, condition. Within the very large and heterogeneous category of consumer-focused health IT, a few have the potential to increase patient engagement in their own health management (see Box 5-1).

To better understand the impact of consumer health IT, the Agency for Healthcare Research and Quality (AHRQ) held a workshop and issued a

---

BOX 5-1
Sample of Consumer Health IT Tools and Services

- Personal health records (integrated and free standing)
- Applications on common devices like smart phones (technology that provides voice and text communication, video and transmission of wireless monitoring data)
- Access to health information (via multiple electronic sources)
- Integration with remote monitoring (personal and home devices and observation systems)
- Internet-based social networking and support
- Internet-based search engines and electronic knowledge bases
- Internet-based administrative services that support care coordination (appointment scheduling, prescription refills, lab results)
- Decision support tools for assessing day-to-day health status or progress toward a health-specific goal (e.g., weight loss, glucose control, caloric intake, cardiac fitness)
- Devices supporting remote monitoring and transmission of data (e.g., from a patient's home environment to a clinician or health "coach")

report in 2010 recognizing that the contribution of consumer health IT to intended and unintended consequences will need to be analyzed continually. The report recommended "[r]igorous research is needed to examine the impact of consumer health IT use on various outcomes (including behavioral, clinical, patient experience, provider experience, efficiency, and unanticipated outcomes), and the specific relationship of design to those outcomes" (Wilson and Peterson, 2010).

PERSONAL HEALTH RECORDS

One tool of particular importance to engage patients and their families is the PHR. PHRs may include features such as health and lifestyle records, ability to book appointments and receive reminders, patient–doctor messaging, and consultation summaries. PHRs are classified as either integrated PHRs or freestanding PHRs. The extent of the differences depends on the specific implementation of the PHR, but this discussion focuses on data and content, stewardship, and self-management features and tools. While considerations of privacy, security, and confidentiality are critical to the development of PHRs, the committee deemed full discussion of these issues to be outside the statement of task.

Data and Content

Integrated PHRs are an essential component of many EHR systems. Data from a resource (e.g., EHRs, insurance claims) populate an integrated PHR. Many of these systems typically offer a portal for secure, online patient access and can serve as an interface to provide useful information to both patients and health professionals. The patient is given a view to key elements of the EHR. In some integrated PHRs, patients can add supplemental data under the broad heading of patient experience, including activities of daily living, reactions to treatments, self-management activities such as exercise, dietary diaries, and data collected from another primary device (e.g., glucometer readings, scales, blood pressure devices). Patients may also amend data, track progress on chronic health issues, and/or otherwise interact with their care team via the portal. Patients can download their PHR to paper or electronic format for transport. While it is difficult to build an integrated PHR that allows health professionals to communicate effectively with their patients, a few EHRs do this well and could serve as models as other products are developed.

Freestanding PHRs such as Microsoft HealthVault are not linked to an EHR, although many of them may allow individuals to access data from different providers' EHRs. Enabling measures such as the "blue button" concept developed by the Markle Foundation (Ellerin Health Media, 2010) could help consumers download electronic copies of health records to a location of their choice; this capability exists with the MyHealtheVet and MyMedicare. They may be especially useful to the health of certain population groups such as migrant workers (MiVia, 2011).

Stewardship

One primary distinction between integrated and freestanding PHRs is that many integrated PHRs do not require patients to actively manage or maintain their data yet still allow access to clinical data. In contrast, the individual (and possibly his legal proxy) is typically primarily responsible for initiating and maintaining all aspects of a freestanding PHR—including collecting, organizing, and storing data—but there are potentially fewer opportunities to validate secondarily or verify the accuracy of content. Thus, the individual patient controls all aspects of the freestanding PHR.

Self-Management Features and Tools

In addition to serving as a repository of personal health data, PHRs may provide patients with other health management and communication tools. Portals within integrated PHRs provide access to records and data, as well as convenience tools for appointments, prescriptions, billing questions, and other communications.

To date, freestanding PHRs have had more limited adoption than integrated PHRs. The future of freestanding PHRs is unclear (Google decided in June 2011 to discontinue marketing and supporting its application Google Health).

MITIGATING SAFETY RISKS OF PATIENT ENGAGEMENT TOOLS: "RULES OF ENGAGEMENT"

The discussion of Chapter 3 introduced the idea of viewing health IT as a component in a larger sociotechnical system that includes technology, people, processes, organizational practices, and the external environment. Adding patients themselves inserts an additional layer of complexity in thinking about how to enhance the safety of patient safety tools in actual use.

For example, although PHRs and other patient engagement tools are designed to have a positive impact on patients' management of their own health, computer-mediated interactions between people are known to be more prone to misinterpretation and misunderstanding than interactions conducted face-to-face (Epley and Kruger, 2005; Kruger et al., 2005). Given the importance of clear patient-provider communications, special attention may have to be devoted to ensuring that computer-mediated interactions are not used inappropriately. Compensation and payment plans and/or job expectations for care providers may have to be adjusted if sufficient amounts of useful information are to be delivered to patients. Freestanding PHRs will need to be designed so that health professionals can track easily and clearly the provenance, accuracy, and currency of data that they did not themselves enter. Health professionals will need to establish procedures to identify and correct errors in an integrated PHR. To be most effective, these mechanisms have to be communicated to patients and their families.

Questions surrounding how PHRs can facilitate communications will require health professionals to manage patient expectations. Health professionals and patients and their families need to develop a shared understanding of appropriate use of patient-entered, validated data. An example of an expectation to be discussed is the types of health problems that are both appropriate and inappropriate for electronic models of communication alone. Managing expectations of both patients and health professionals as to the currency of information and the turnaround time for various applications can have implications for patient safety.

PHRs and other patient engagement tools will benefit from employing user-centered design that enhances the ability of patients and their families to take part in their care management and coordination. There is growing interest in providing mechanisms that support patient and family feedback to providers and clinicians about their experiences of care so as to inform safety and quality improvement. Innovative and flexible applications offer greater opportunity for engagement (Brennan et al., 2010). Features might include using general IT solutions familiar to patients and their families (both non-Internet-based and Internet-based). Simple, easy data entry ought to be available through a variety of different means (e.g., touch interface, key strokes, mouse). Common international standards for such patient applications may reduce confusion and support both utilization and safe use. An international team has developed a global EHR template standard for PHRs that offers patients the flexibility of the record summary remaining on the web, being stored in a cell phone, being used on a computer, or being stored on a flash drive (Li et al., 2012). Such a ubiquitous standard for data structure and minimal EHR elements offers an excellent research opportunity for greater use and also safety studies.

Use of mobile applications (mobile apps) has become more widespread and a wide variety of mobile medical apps has been developed. As of July 2011, the Food and Drug Administration (FDA) has issued draft guidance stating that it will only regulate mobile applications that either impact the performance or functionality of currently regulated medical devices or have conventionally been considered medical devices. These apps will be classified and regulated similarly to other medical devices under FDA's jurisdiction. Apps to be used as PHRs, to track general health and wellness such as dietary logs and calorie counters, and to automate common medical knowledge will only be regulated at FDA's discretion (FDA, 2011). As new apps are developed that serve patients and their families as a mobile medical device, their impact on safety will need to be examined.

It is important to note that, although not directly related to safety, over-reliance on technology as a vehicle to provide patients access to their health data or other decision-making tools may create barriers for many consumers. Limited access by some populations as a result of the availability of hardware and high-speed Internet connectivity may diminish broad access and create inequities or exacerbate disparities. Furthermore, obtaining the knowledge and skills needed to navigate the Internet, sign up for portal access, and then use the sites effectively may be intimidating, challenging, or impossible for some patients. English-language proficiency, health literacy levels, and numeracy skills all play important roles in the ability of an individual to interpret, understand, and use most of the data and information stored in electronic records, much as in paper records (Yamin et al., 2011).

POPULATION HEALTH MANAGEMENT

Technologies are emerging that will enhance tracking of population health. Reporting of conditions to health departments, and recording emergency and natural disaster situations, can inform community and public health officials about health and illness patterns and needs. Populating databases about lifestyle, healthy behaviors, and disease prevention interventions will add new knowledge to our system that currently focuses mainly on diseases and treatment. As data are analyzed across communities, workers and clinicians can learn about local health risks and disease rates. In addition to reporting and querying information, core functionalities of a population health record would include generating alerts, identifying disease outbreaks and trends, identifying geographic influences on illness, and reporting of behaviors impacting health or development of disease (Friedman and Parrish, 2010). Longitudinal records can bring together data from PHRs, EHRs, and public health agencies. Eventually, analysis of health care equity across populations may guide approaches to eliminate health disparities.

PHRs can boost patient safety not only at the individual level but also for aggregate populations. Accessing patient information across care settings is essential to future enhancements in safe delivery of care (Kilbridge and Classen, 2008). As communities promote nationwide exchange of health information, pooling of information about consumer engagement and learning strategies can reveal approaches for better integration of PHRs with provider records and engagement of consumers in health-promoting behaviors.

CONCLUSION

The field of patient engagement tools that rely on health IT is rapidly developing and offers many potential benefits to patient care. However, the unintended consequences these tools may have, such as threats to patient safety, have not been adequately studied. The increasing use of health IT by consumers, patients, and families creates an urgent need for the development and support of a research agenda to inform future public policy about the design, implementation, and use of such tools.

REFERENCES

Brennan, P. F., S. Downs, and G. Casper. 2010. Project HealthDesign: Rethinking the power and potential of personal health records. *Journal of Biomedical Informatics* 43(5 Suppl 1):S3-S5.

California HealthCare Foundation. 2010. *Consumers and health information technology: A survey.* Oakland, CA.

Detmer, D., M. Bloomrosen, B. Raymond, and P. Tang. 2008. Integrated personal health records: Transformative tools for consumer-centric care. *BMC Medical Informatics and Decision Making* 8:45.

Ellerin Health Media. 2010. *Markle Foundation and the blue button.* http://ellerinhealthmedia. com/2010/10/19/markle-foundation-and-the-blue-button/ (accessed June 27, 2011).

Epley, N., and J. Kruger. 2005. When what you type isn't what they read: The perseverance of stereotypes and expectancies over e-mail. *Journal of Experimental Social Psychology* 41:414-422.

FDA (Food and Drug Adminisitration). 2011. *Draft guidance for industry and Food and Drug Administration staff—mobile medical applications.*

Fricton, J. R., and D. Davies. 2008. Personal health records to improve health information exchange and patient safety technology and medication safety. In *Advances in patient safety: New directions and alternative approaches*, Vol. 4. Rockville, MD: Agency for Healthcare Research and Quality.

Friedman, D. J., and R. G. Parrish. 2010. The population health record: Concepts, definition, design, and implementation. *Journal of the American Medical Informatics Association* 17(4):359-366.

Gandhi, T. K., S. N. Weingart, J. Borus, A. C. Seger, J. Peterson, E. Burdick, D. L. Seger, K. Shu, F. Federico, L. L. Leape, and D.W. Bates. 2003. Adverse drug events in ambulatory care. *New England Journal of Medicine* 348(16):1556-1564.

HHS (Department of Health and Human Services). 2011. *Report to Congress: National strategy for quality improvement in health care.* http://www.healthcare.gov/center/reports/ quality03212011a.html#es (accessed June 27, 2011).

IOM (Institute of Medicine). 2001. *Crossing the quality chasm: A new health system for the 21st century.* Washington, DC: National Academy Press.

Kilbridge, P. M., and D. C. Classen. 2008. The informatics opportunities at the intersection of patient safety and clinical informatics. *Journal of the American Medical Informatics Association* 15(4):397-407.

Kruger, J., N. Epley, J. Parker, Z. Ng. 2005. Egocentrism over e-mail: Can we communicate as well as we think? *Journal of Personality and Social Psychology* 89(6):925-936.

Li, Y., D. Detmer, S. Shabbir, P. A. Nguyen, W. Jian, G. I. Mihalas, E. H. Shortliffe, P. Tang, R. Haux, M. Kirmura, and K. Toyoda. 2012. A global travelers' electronic health record template (TrEHRT) standard for personal health records. *Journal of the American Medical Informatics Association* 19(1):134-136.

MiVia. 2011. *About MiVia.* https://www.mivia.org/about_us.aspx (accessed June 27, 2011).

NQF (National Quality Forum). 2011. *National priorities partnership: Priorities.* http://www.nationalprioritiespartnership.org/PriorityDetails.aspx?id=596 (accessed July 30, 2011).

ONC (Office of the National Coordinator for Health Information Technology). 2011. *Health IT strategic plan 2011-2015.* http://healthit.hhs.gov/portal/server.pt?open=512&objID=1211&parentname=CommunityPage&parentid=2&mode=2 (accessed June 27, 2011).

Patel, V. N., R. V. Dhopeshwarkar, A. Edwards, Y. Barron, J. Sparenborg, and R. Kaushal. 2010. Consumer support for health information exchange and personal health records: A regional health information organization survey. *Journal of Medical Systems* (July 29, 2011 [Epub ahead of print]).

PCAST (President's Council of Advisors on Science and Technology). 2010. *Realizing the full potential of health information technology to improve healthcare for Americans: The path forward.* http://www.whitehouse.gov/sites/default/files/microsites/ostp/pcast-health-it-report.pdf (accessed May 18, 2011).

Pew Research Center. 2011. *Health topics.* http://www.pewinternet.org/~/media/Files/Reports/2011/PIP_HealthTopics.pdf (accessed August 9, 2011).

Poon, E. G., J. Wald, J. L. Schnipper, R. Grant, T. K. Gandhi, L. A. Volk, A. Bloom, D. H. Williams, K. Gardner, M. Epstein, L. Nelson, A. Businger, Q. Li, D. W. Bates, and B. Middleton. 2007. Empowering patients to improve the quality of their care: Design and implementation of a shared health maintenance module in a US integrated healthcare delivery network. *Studies in Health Technology and Informatics* 129(Pt 2):1002-1006.

Skorve, E. 2010. Patient safety, resilience and ICT. A reason for concern? *Studies in Health Technology and Informatics* 157:199-205.

Wen, K. Y., G. Kreps, F. Zhu, and S. Miller. 2010. Consumers' perceptions about and use of the Internet for personal health records and health information exchange: Analysis of the 2007 Health Information National Trends Survey. *Journal of Medical Internet Research* 12(4):e73-e73.

Wilson, C., and A. Peterson. 2010. *Managing personal health information: An action agenda.* Rockville, MD: Agency for Healthcare Research and Quality.

Yamin, C. K., S. Emani, D. H. Williams, S. R. Lipsitz, A. S. Karson, J. S. Wald, and D. W. Bates. 2011. The digital divide in adoption and use of a personal health record. *Archives of Internal Medicine* 171(6):568-574.

Zhou, Y., M. H. Kanter, J. J. Wang, and T. Garrido. 2010. Improved qualilty at Kaiser Permanente through e-mail between physicians and patients. *Health Affairs* 29(7):1370-1375.

6

A Shared Responsibility for Improving Health IT Safety

As discussed in Chapter 2, the use of health IT in some areas has significantly improved the quality of health care and reduced medical errors. Continuing to use paper medical records can place patients at unnecessary risk for harm and substantially constrain the country's ability to reform the health care system. However, there are clearly cases in which harm has occurred associated with new health IT. The committee believes safer health care is possible in complex, dynamic environments—which are the rule in health care—only when achieving and maintaining safety is given a high priority.

Achieving the desired reduction in harm will depend on a number of factors, including how the technology is designed, how it is implemented, how well it fits into clinical workflow, how it supports informed decision making by both patients and providers, and whether it is safe and reliable. An environment of safer health IT can be created if both the public and private sectors acknowledge that safety is a shared responsibility. Actions are needed to correct the market and commit to ensuring the safety of health IT. A better understanding and acknowledgement of the risks associated with health IT and its use, as well as how to maximize the benefits, are needed. An example of a new kind of error that can occur with IT which did not occur previously is the "adjacency error," in which a provider selects an item next to the one intended from a pulldown menu, for example picking "penicillamine" instead of "penicillin." Such errors occur in many products, but effective solutions have not yet generally been fielded. This chapter details the actions to be taken by both the public and private sectors that the committee believes will be necessary for the creation of an environment in which IT improves safety overall, and the new problems created by health IT are minimized.

THE ROLE OF THE PRIVATE SECTOR: PROMOTING SHARED LEARNING ENVIRONMENTS

This chapter broadly defines the private sector to include health IT vendors, insurers, and the organizations that support each of these groups (e.g., professional societies). Health care organizations, health professionals, and patients and their families are also considered part of the private sector. The public sector generally refers to the government. Operationally, the line between the private and public sectors is not completely clear, because some organizations operate in both sectors.

The current environment in which health IT is designed and used does not adequately protect patient safety. However, the private sector has the ability to drive innovation and creativity, generating the tools to deliver the best possible health care and directly improve safety. In this regard, the private sector has the most direct responsibility to realign the market, but it will need support from the public sector.

The complexity and dynamism of health IT requires that private-sector entities work together through shared learning to improve patient safety. Manufacturers and health professionals have to communicate their capabilities and needs to each other to facilitate the design of health IT in ways that achieve maximum usability and safety. Patients and their families need to be able to interact seamlessly with health professionals through patient engagement tools. Health care organizations ought to share lessons learned with each other to avoid common patient safety risks as they adopt highly complex health IT products.

However, today's reality is that the private sector currently consists of a broad variety of stakeholders lacking a uniform approach, and potentially misaligned goals. The track record of the private sector in responding to new safety issues created by IT is mixed. Although nearly all stakeholders would endorse the broad goals of improving the quality and safety of patient care, many stakeholders (particularly vendors) are faced with competing priorities, including maximizing profits and maintaining a competitive edge, which can limit shared learning, and have adverse consequences for patient safety. Shared learning about safety risks and mitigation strategies for safer health IT among users, vendors, researchers, and other stakeholders, can optimize patient safety and minimize harm.

As discussed in Chapters 4 and 5, there are many opportunities for the private sector to improve safety as it relates to health IT, but to date, little action has been taken. Insufficient action by the private sector to improve patient safety can endanger lives. The private sector must play a major role in addressing this urgent need to better understand risks and benefits associated with health IT, as well as strategies for improvement and remediation. As it stands now, there is a lack of accountability on the part of vendors, who are generally perceived to shift responsibility and accountability to users through specific contract language (Goodman et al., 2010). As a result, the committee believes a number of critical gaps in knowledge need to be addressed immediately, including the lack of comprehensive mechanisms for identifying patient safety risks, measuring health IT safety, ensuring safe implementation, and educating and training users.

Developing a System for Identifying Patient Safety Risks

The committee believes that transparency, characterized by developing, identifying, and sharing evidence on risks to patient safety, is essential to a properly functioning market where users would have the ability to choose a product that best suits their needs and the needs of their patients. However, the committee found sparse evidence pertaining to the volume and types of patient safety risks related to health IT. Indeed, the number of errors reported both anecdotally and in the published literature was lower than the committee anticipated. This led primarily to the sense that potentially harmful situations and adverse events caused by IT were often not recognized and, even when they were recognized, usually not reported. This lack of reported instances of harm is consistent with other areas of patient safety, including paper-based patient records and other manually based care systems, where there is ample evidence that most adverse events are never reported, even when there are robust programs encouraging health professionals to do so (Classen et al., 2011; Cullen et al., 1995).

Information technology can assist organizations in identifying, troubleshooting, and handling health IT–related adverse events. Digital forensic tools (e.g., centralized logging, regular system backups) can be used to record data during system use. After an adverse event occurs, recorded data—such as log-in information, keystrokes, and how information is transported throughout the network—can be used to identify, reconstruct, and understand in detail how an adverse event occurred (NIST, 2006).

Because of the diversity of health IT products and their differing effects on various clinical environments, it is essential that users share detailed information with other users, researchers, and the vendor once information regarding adverse events is identified. Examples of such information include screenshots or descriptions of potentially unsafe processes that could help illustrate how a health IT product threatened patient safety. However, as discussed in Chapter 2, users may fear that sharing this information may violate nondisclosure clauses and vendors' intellectual property, exposing them to liability and litigation. Although there is little evidence on the impact of such clauses, the committee believes users may be less likely to share information necessary to improve patient safety, given these clauses.

If it is clearly understood that transparently sharing health IT issues with the public is for the purpose of patient safety, vendors ought to agree to remove such restrictions from contracts and work with users to explicitly define what can be shared, who it can be shared with, and for what purposes. However, to maintain a competitive advantage, many vendors may not be motivated to allow users to disclose patient safety–related risks associated with their health IT products. Many vendors place these clauses within the boilerplate language, and in the absence of comprehensive legal review, users may not even realize these restrictions exist when signing their contracts.[1] If more users carefully search for such clauses and negotiate terms that allow them to share information related to patient safety risks, vendors may be more likely to exclude such clauses. Furthermore, if it were easier to know which vendors had standard contracts that allowed for sharing, users might be more likely to select those vendors. However, users—particularly smaller organizations—are not part of a "cohesive community" with the legal expertise or knowledge to negotiate such changes. Therefore, the committee believes the Secretary of the Department of Health and Human Services (HHS) should provide tools to motivate vendors and empower users to negotiate contracts that allow for sharing of patient safety–related details and improved transparency. The Secretary ought to investigate what other tools and authorities would be required to ensure the free exchange of patient safety–related information.

> **Recommendation 2: The Secretary of HHS should ensure insofar as possible that health IT vendors support the free exchange of information about health IT experiences and issues and not prohibit sharing of such information, including details (e.g., screenshots) relating to patient safety.**

The committee recognizes that, short of Congressional and regulatory action, the Secretary cannot guarantee how contracts are developed between two private parties. However, the committee views prohibition of the free exchange of information to be the most critical barrier to patient safety and transparency. The committee urges the Secretary to take vigorous steps to restrict contractual language that impedes public sharing of patient safety–related details. Contracts should be developed to allow explicitly for sharing of health IT issues related to patient safety. One method the Secretary could use is to ask the Office of the National Coordinator for Health Information Technology (ONC) to create a list of vendors that satisfy this

---

[1] Personal communication, E. Belmont, MaineHealth, September 21, 2011.

requirement and/or those that do not. If such a list were available, users could more easily choose vendors that allow patient safety–related details of health IT products to be shared. Having such a list could also motivate vendors to include contractual terms that allow for sharing of patient safety–related details and, as a result, be more competitive to users. The ONC could also consider creating minimum criteria for determining when a contract adequately allows for sharing of patient safety–related details. These criteria need to define the following:

- What situations allow for sharing patient safety–related details of health IT products;
- What content of health IT should be shareable;
- Which stakeholders the information can be shared with, including other users, consumer groups, researchers, and the government; and
- What the limitations of liability are when such information is shared.

Private certification bodies such as the ONC-authorized testing and certification bodies (ONC-ATCBs)[2] could also promote the free exchange of patient safety-related information. This could be implemented for example through the creation of a new type of certification that requires this information to be shared.

The Secretary could ask the ONC to develop model contract language that would affirmatively establish the ability of users to provide content and contextual information when reporting an adverse event or unsafe condition. Additionally, HHS could educate users about these contracts and develop guidance for users about what to look for before signing a contract. This education could potentially be done through the ONC's regional extension centers or the Centers for Medicare & Medicaid Services's (CMS's) quality improvement organizations. This effort could also be supported by various professional societies.

To identify how pervasive these clauses are, the Secretary may need to conduct a review of existing contracts. Although the Secretary may not be privy to vendor–purchaser contracts, HHS could conduct a survey or ask vendors to voluntarily share examples of their contract language. Understanding the magnitude of these clauses would be a critical first step.

Once this information is available, comparative user experiences can be made public. There is currently no effective way for users to communicate their experiences with a health IT product. In many other industries, user

---

[2] ONC-ATCBs as of April 2011 include the Certification Commission for Health Information Technology; Drummond Group, Inc.; ICSALabs; InfoGard Laboratories, Inc.; SLI Globan Solutions; and Surescripts LLC.

reviews appear on online forums and other similar guides, while independent tests are conducted by Consumer Reports and others. These reviews allow users to better understand the products they might be purchasing. Perhaps the more powerful aspect of users being able to rate and compare their experiences with products is the ability to share and report lessons learned. Comparative user experiences for health IT safety need to be created to enhance communication of safety concerns and ways to mitigate potential risks.

To gather objective information about health IT products, researchers should have access to both test versions of software provided by vendors and software already integrated in user organizations. Documentation for health IT products such as user manuals also could be made available to researchers. Resources should be available to share user experiences and other measures of safety specifying data from health IT products. The private sector needs to be a catalyzing force in this area, but governance from the public sector may be required for such tools to be developed.

Recommendation 3: The ONC should work with the private and public sectors to make comparative user experiences across vendors publicly available.

Another way to increase transparency in the private sector is to require reporting of health IT–related adverse events through health care provider accrediting organizations such as The Joint Commission or the National Committee for Quality Assurance (NCQA). Professional associations of providers could also play this role. One of the tools the ONC could provide to facilitate the implementation of Recommendation 3 is the development of a uniform format for making these reports, which could be coordinated through the Common Formats.[3] However, it is important to note that a public-sector entity could also lead change in this regard.

Finally, a more robust and comprehensive infrastructure is needed for providing technical assistance to users who may need advice or training to safely implement health IT products. Shared learning between users and vendors in the form of feedback about how well health IT products are working can help improve the focus on safety and usability in the design of health IT products and identification of performance requirements. Tools to foster this feedback in an organized way are needed to promote safety and quality. The learning curve for safely using health IT–assisted care varies widely and technical assistance needs to be provided to users at all levels.

---

[3] The Common Formats are coordinated by the Agency for Healthcare Research and Quality (AHRQ) in an effort to facilitate standardized reporting of adverse events by creating general definitions and reporting formats for widespread use (AHRQ, 2011a).

Measuring Health IT Safety

Another area the committee identified as necessary for making health IT safer is the development of measures. As is often said in quality improvement, you can only improve what you measure. Currently, few measures address patient safety as it relates to health IT; without these measures, it will be very difficult to develop and test strategies to ensure safe patient care. Although there has been progress in developing general measures of patient safety, the committee concluded that safety measures focusing on the impact of health IT must go beyond traditional safety measures (as discussed in Chapter 3) and are urgently needed.

Measures of health care safety and quality are generally developed by groups such as professional societies and academic researchers and undergo a voluntary consensus process before being adopted for widespread use. During the measure development process, decisions need to be made such as identifying what metrics can be used as an indicator of health IT safety, specifications of the metrics, and the criteria against which measures can be evaluated. Policies for measure ownership and processes for evaluating and maintaining measures will also need to be created. One example of the type of data that are likely to be important would be override rates for important types of safety warnings on alerts and warnings built into electronic health records (EHRs).

The committee believes a consensus-based collaborative effort that would oversee development, application, and evaluation of criteria for measures and best practices of safety of health IT—a Health IT Safety Council—is of vital need. For example, the council could be responsible for identifying key performance aspects of health IT and creating a prioritized agenda for measure development. Given that the process for developing health IT safety metrics would be similar to developing measures of health care safety and quality, a voluntary consensus standards organization would effectively be able to house the recommended council. Because of the ubiquity and complexity of health IT, all health IT stakeholders ought to be involved in the development of such criteria. HHS ought to consider providing the initial funding for the council because the need for measures of safety of health IT is central to all stakeholders. The more costly process of maintaining measures ought to be funded by private-sector entities.

Recommendation 4: The Secretary of HHS should fund a new Health IT Safety Council to evaluate criteria for assessing and monitoring the safe use of health IT and the use of health IT to enhance safety. This council should operate within an existing voluntary consensus standards organization.

One existing organization with a strong history of convening groups and experience with endorsing health care quality and performance measures that could guide this process is the National Quality Forum (NQF). The NQF is a nonprofit organization whose mission is to develop consensus on national priorities and endorse standards for measuring and publicly reporting on health care performance based on measures submitted from measure developers. Of particular note, the NQF hosts eight member councils, whose purposes are to build consensus among council members toward advancing quality measurement and reporting (NQF, 2011). These councils provide a voice to stakeholder groups—including consumers, health professionals, health care organizations, professional organizations (e.g., the American Medical Informatics Association [AMIA]), vendors (e.g., individually and through societies such as the Healthcare Information and Management Systems Society [HIMSS]), and insurers—to identify what types of metrics are needed and the criteria for doing so. Measures should be NQF-endorsed, a process that applies nationally accepted standards and criteria. The NQF could provide guidance in identifying criteria against which to develop health IT safety measures to help gain consensus on the right set of policies.

The ensuing task of developing measures of health IT safety needs to be undertaken by a variety of entities. To accomplish this, some research will be needed for measure development because good measures currently do not exist; these efforts should be supported by the Agency for Healthcare Research and Quality (AHRQ), the National Library of Medicine, and the ONC, as discussed in Recommendation 1. Health care organizations and even vendors could partner with more traditional measurement development organizations, for example the NCQA can create measures that would by default be subjected to the NQF consensus approval process.

Ensuring Safer Implementation

Efforts to safely implement health IT must address three phases: preimplementation, implementation, and postimplementation of health IT.

Preimplementation

Vendors, with input from users, play the most significant role in the preimplementation phase of health IT. Vendors ought to be able to assert that their products are designed and developed in a way that promotes patient safety. Currently, health IT products are held to few standards with respect to both design and development. Although it is typically the role of standards development organizations such as the American National Standards Institute, the Association for the Advancement of Medical Instrumentation, Health Level 7 (HL7), and the Institute of Electrical and Electronics

Engineers to develop such standards, criteria, and tests, a broader group of stakeholders including patients, users, and vendors should participate in creating safety standards and criteria against which health IT ought to be tested.

Vendors are currently being required by the ONC to meet a specific set of criteria in order for their products to be certified as eligible for use in HHS's meaningful use program. These criteria relate to clinical functionality, security, and interoperability and may be helpful for but not sufficient to ensure health IT–related safety. The American National Standards Institute, as the body that will accredit organizations that certify health IT, and certification bodies such as the Certification Commission for Healthcare Information Technology serve a vital function in this regard because they have the ability to require that patient safety be an explicit criterion for certification of EHRs. Doing so would be an important first step.

Another step that can be taken by the private sector prior to implementation of health IT is for vendors and manufacturers to declare they have addressed safety issues in the design and development of their products, both self-identified issues and those detected during product testing. Such a declaration ought to include the safety issues considered and the steps taken to address those issues. A similar declaration for usability has been supported by the National Institute of Standards and Technology (NIST), which has developed a common industry format for health IT manufacturers to declare that they have tested their products for usability and asks manufacturers to show evidence of usability (NIST, 2010). Declarations also ought to be made with respect to vendor tests of a health IT product's reliability and response time, both in vitro and in situ (Sittig and Classen, 2010). Such declarations could provide users and purchasers of health IT with information as they determine which products to acquire. Additionally, vendors can help mitigate safety risks by employing high-quality software engineering principles, as discussed in Chapter 4.

Usability represents an exceptionally important issue overall, and undoubtedly affects safety. However, it would be challenging to mandate usability. Although some efforts are beginning to develop usability standards and tools as discussed in Chapter 4, more publicly available data about and testing regarding usability would be helpful in this area. EHRs should increasingly use standards and conformance testing to ensure that data from EHRs meet certain standards and would be readable by other systems to enable interoperability is practical.

Besides providing feedback to vendors about their products, users also have important responsibilities for safety during the preimplementation phase. Users need to make the often difficult and nuanced decision of choosing a product to purchase, as discussed in Chapter 4. If a product does not meet the needs of the organization and does not appropriately interface with other IT products of the organization, safety problems can arise. Similarly, organizations need to be ready to adopt a new product in order for the transition to be successful.

Implementation

Industry-developed recommended (or "best") practices and lessons learned ought to be shared. There are instances where generic lessons are learned and recommended practices can be shared between health professionals through mediums such as forums, chat rooms, and conferences. Lessons can also be shared through training opportunities such as continuing professional development activities. Questions arise such as whether to roll out a health IT product throughout an entire health care organization at once or in parts. Health care providers are continually attempting to determine the most effective configuration of health IT products for their own specific situations (e.g., drug interactions should be displayed as warnings in such a way that clinicians do not suffer from alert fatigue, leading clinicians to turn off all alerts). A user's guide to acquisition and implementation ought to be developed by both the private and public sectors. Some efforts are currently under way, including programs at HIMSS and the ONC, but more work is needed, and the committee believes that such user's guides should receive public support, though they might be developed by private entities.

Opportunities also exist for users to learn more about safer implementation and customization of health IT products. For example, what lessons have been learned regarding customization of specific health IT products? What experiences have others had integrating a specific pharmacy system with a particular EHR? Lessons from such experiences, once they are widely shared, can greatly impact implementation. It will be critical for users and vendors to communicate as health IT products are being implemented to ensure they are functioning correctly and are fitting into clinical workflow.

Postimplementation

Similar to the preimplementation and implementation phases, standards and criteria will be necessary to ensure that users have appropriately implemented health IT products and integrated them into the entire sociotechnical system. In the postimplementation phase, the largest share of the work involves health professionals and organizations working with vendors to ensure patient safety.

Postimplementation tests, as discussed in Chapter 4, will be essential to monitoring the successful implementation of health IT products. Few tests currently exist, and more will need to be developed. For example, self-assessments could monitor the product's down time, review the ability to perform common actions (e.g., review recent lab results), and record patient safety events. Ongoing tests of how the product is operating with respect to the full sociotechnical system could identify areas for improvement to ensure the product fits into the clinical workflow safely and effectively (Classen and Bates, 2011; Sittig and Classen, 2010; Sittig and Singh, 2009). These tests are also a way for users to work with vendors to ensure that products have been installed correctly. Developers of these postimplementation tests should gather input from health care organizations, clinicians, vendors, and the general public. Similar to how organizations such as the Leapfrog Group validate tests for effective implementation of computerized provider order entry systems, an independent group ought to validate test results for implementation of all health IT. Conducting these tests is so important for ensuring safety that they ought to become a required standard and linked to a health care organization's accreditation through The Joint Commission or others. Periodic inspections could also be conducted onsite by these external accreditation organizations (Sittig and Classen, 2010). Other ways to require these tests be performed include actions from the public sector, including regulation, such as including postimplementation testing in meaningful use criteria, but the committee feels postimplementation testing is too important to be tied only to the initiatives of a particular government program. These issues of safer implementation and safer use will continue to be an ongoing challenge with each new iteration of software and will continue to be an important area of focus long after the meaningful use program is completed.

Training Professionals to Use Health IT Safely

Education and training of the workforce is critical to the successful adoption of change. If the workforce is not educated and trained correctly, workers will be less likely to use health IT as effectively as their properly trained counterparts. Educating health professionals about health IT and safety can help them understand the complexities of health IT from the perspective of the sociotechnical system. This allows health professionals to transfer context- and product-specific skills, and therefore to be safer and more effective. For example, a team of clinicians using a new electronic pharmacy system needs to be trained on the functionalities of the specific technology. Otherwise, the team is susceptible either to being naïve to the abilities of the technology or to unnecessarily developing workarounds that may undermine the larger sociotechnical system.

As discussed in earlier chapters, basic levels of competence, knowledge, and skill are needed to navigate the highly complex implementation of health IT. Because health IT exists at the intersection of multiple disciplines, a variety of professionals will need training in this relatively new discipline that builds off the established fields of health systems, IT, and clinical care (Gardner et al., 2009). Training in the unique knowledge of health IT will be important, particularly for organizational leadership, IT professionals, and health professionals.

Organizational Leadership

Often it is the leadership of a health care organization that makes decisions about the various types of technologies to acquire based on the needs of the clinicians and patients. However, the decisions related to acquiring health IT are more complicated than acquiring other types of technologies such as computed tomography scanners and magnetic resonance imaging machines and require a specific body of knowledge. In order to select the most appropriate health IT product and make informed decisions, organizational leaders will need to be aware of specific considerations, such as whether to implement a health IT product all at once or in a sequential fashion, whether the vendor or the organization should be responsible for backing up data, and whether the health IT product will need to be interoperable with other products already in place, both internal and external to the organization. Understanding the issues related to health IT and its potential effects on patient safety is critical because of the large investment and continued resources needed for safer, more effective implementation of health IT.

The role of the chief medical and/or nursing information officer has been designed to be vital to the success of health IT, serving as a bridge between IT staff and clinicians. Small practices may relate to local hospitals or assign someone within their office, whether a clinician or not, to help lead these efforts. For example, the Chief Medical Information Officer Bootcamp offered by AMIA and tutorials or program offerings by organizations such as AMIA, the American Medical Directors of Information Systems, the College of Healthcare Information Management Executives, and the Scottsdale Institute can help identify and train appropriate personnel. Additionally, a better connection between the clinical informatics community and medical and nursing specialty society organizations would be helpful, such as the chief nursing information officers link promoted by HIMSS. Appointing a chief medical and/or nursing information officer allows for health care organizations to hold someone accountable for the implementation and use of health IT. As discussed in Chapter 3, truly being able to use health IT products and ensuring their safety requires a unique set of skills.

IT Professionals

With respect to the implementation and maintenance of technologies, a growing number of IT professionals are being trained to work with clinicians to redesign workflow as well as to manage and support implementation of health IT. The ONC supports a workforce development program to provide training at these levels. In May 2011, the ONC released a series of health IT competency exams for individual health IT professionals to demonstrate their knowledge level in acquiring health IT products, implementing and maintaining them, and training other staff on how to use them (ONC, 2011). IT professionals provide a key support function in health IT–enabled care delivery and therefore need to be trained on clinical workflows to best support clinicians and understand why workarounds that can lead to unsafe care are developed.

Health Professionals

While health professionals are rarely specialists in technologies themselves, they bear arguably the greatest responsibility for daily use of the technology and likely feel substantial responsibility to ensure that health IT products are not harmful to their patients. To optimize the potential for health IT to improve the safety of patient care, health professionals must not only learn how to use specific health IT products and about their full functionality but also learn how to incorporate these products into their daily workflows. If not properly trained on how to use a specific technology, health professionals may not only miss an opportunity to make their own processes safer and more efficient, but also may in fact develop unsafe conditions. At a minimum, clinicians need to be trained to recognize that health IT can improve quality of care while being cognizant of its potential to negatively impact patient safety if used inappropriately.

To date, programs focusing on training health professionals to use health IT generally are not widespread. As part of the ONC's health IT workforce development program, health professionals can learn techniques related to implementation. Although this is a step in the right direction, other, more specific and comprehensive programs are needed to complement this training that focus more specifically on using health IT and to do so in an interprofessional manner. The opportunity to provide care in interprofessional teams and improve communications may be essential to providing safer care, shifting the paradigm of health care delivery. In addition to the fact that almost all health IT products are configured differently, health professionals' interaction with IT products differs by specialty, by profession, by health care setting, and even by state.

Clinician education and training can be encouraged through a number of avenues, including formal education and postgraduate training as well as the longer course of clinicians' careers. Introducing concepts of health IT safety early in professional clinical training (e.g., professional school, residencies) allows clinicians the opportunity to learn how to use and practice delivery of care safely and effectively with a technology in place. As future generations of health professionals grow up using these technologies, they will be more adept at using them on a daily basis throughout their careers. It is also important to be trained in a local context (e.g., by hospital, clinic, nursing home). AMIA has had a program identified as "10×10" to offer rigorous graduate training–level introductory courses in clinical informatics, of which safety is generally a part. Further dissemination and offering of these courses could result in important advances.

AMIA, in partnership with the Robert Wood Johnson Foundation, has also developed a clinical informatics subspecialty through the American Board of Medical Specialties. Many boards are beginning to require a facility with health IT as part of a clinician's maintenance of certification. Some specialty societies such as the American College of Physicians, the American Academy of Pediatrics, and the American College of Surgeons have active informatics committees that could explicitly take up the issue of safety, for discussions relating to both problems and solutions as well as creating a wider array of educational offerings.

To varying degrees, hospitals and other health care organizations require health professionals to be able to use health IT. For example, they often require clinicians to receive a certain number of hours of introduction to the health IT product before granting privileges.

Health IT can facilitate communication in team-based care. As a result, a focus on health IT safety is needed in interdisciplinary settings. An interdisciplinary focus on health IT safety that includes a variety of professionals is essential to safer, widespread use of health IT. A number of organizations are currently focusing on interdisciplinary team training. Nursing groups such as the Alliance for Nursing Informatics, the American Association of Colleges of Nursing, the National League for Nursing, and the American Organization of Nurse Executives are engaging in informatics and ought to continue developing concerted efforts to include safety issues in nursing programs. In addition, the Quality and Safety Education for Nursing program funded by the Robert Wood Johnson Foundation has developed a nursing curriculum that includes pathways for developing knowledge, skills, and attitudes related to patient safety and informatics (Quality and Safety Education for Nurses, 2011). Similar programs focusing on pharmacy training are also under way. For example, the American Society for Health-System Pharmacists has a membership section for pharmacy informatics and technology that sponsors educational programs at their annual meetings. An increasing number of institutions have postgraduate pharmacy informatics specialty residency programs. The leading national pharmacy societies have formed the Pharmacy e-Health Information Technology Collaborative, for which training is a foundational goal. Other health professionals such as physician assistants and physical therapists also need training on health IT, some of which already have efforts under way. Health care executives through organizations such as the American College of Physician Executives also ought to be involved in these efforts.

Most of the foregoing comments relate to education more than simply training, especially with regard to the proper use of specific EHR products and systems. However, training is just as critical to safe use as education and is necessary for users to become aware of limitations of the software and also potential problems that have arisen elsewhere. Hospitals typically have training programs and labs available for clinicians to "dry run" the product and dedicated staff on wards or in clinics to serve as resources for others. Training sessions may be few or many. With specific attention to safety, staff need to know how the software deals with updates, for example drug–drug interactions. Greater attention to the creation of training modules focused on safety is needed, particularly on the strengths and weaknesses of both the software and the institution with respect to its early use of the system.

The committee believes it is incumbent on all stakeholders to participate in the creation of shared learning environments. It is also important to realize that the goal is not only learning by individuals but equally, if not more importantly, learning by the system itself. Through shared learning, health IT products can adapt to new challenges and opportunities while becoming safer over time.

THE ROLE OF THE PUBLIC SECTOR: STRATEGIC GUIDANCE AND OVERSIGHT

The first four recommendations are intended to encourage the private sector to create an environment that facilitates understanding of the risk, gathers data, and promotes change. But in some instances, the private sector cannot create this environment itself. The government in some cases is the only body able to provide policy guidance and direction to complement, bolster, and support private-sector efforts and to correct misaligned market forces. While a bottom-up approach may yield some improvements in safety, it is limited in its breadth. Gaps will arise that require a more comprehensive approach, for example, ensuring processes are in place to report, investigate, and make recommendations to mitigate unsafe conditions associated with health IT–related incidents. This section addresses solutions to some of these gaps.

The Health Information Technology for Economic and Clinical Health legislation has embarked the nation upon a $30 billion investment that will impact both technology and clinical practice on a scale heretofore unseen in the nation (Laflamme et al., 2010). However, it is unclear what value the nation is receiving for its investment. Thus, the public sector has a responsibility to monitor and assess its investment and ensure that it is not harmful to patients. The ONC, AHRQ, the CMS, the National Institutes of Health, the Food and Drug Administration (FDA), and NIST, among other federal agencies, are becoming more actively involved in guiding the future direction of health IT, indicating that patient safety will also require a shared responsibility among federal agencies. However, currently funded government programs are just one part of a multifaceted solution to improving patient safety and health IT.

An appropriate balance must be reached between government oversight or regulation and market innovation. As with most rapidly developing technologies, governmental involvement has the potential to both foster and stifle innovation (Grabowski and Vernon, 1977; Hauptman and Roberts, 1987; Walshe and Shortell, 2004). For example, blood banking has been regulated for some time, and many believe regulation has limited innovation in this domain (Gastineau, 2004; Kim, 2002; Schneider, 1996; Weeda and O'Flaherty, 1998). Stringent regulations, while intended to promote safety, can negatively impact the development of new technology (Grabowski and Vernon, 1977) by limiting implementation choices and restricting manufacturers' flexibility to address complex issues (Cohen, 1979; Marcus, 1988) and may even adversely affect safety. However, regulations also have the potential to increase innovations (see Appendix D) and improve patient safety, especially if manufacturers are not adequately addressing specific safety-related issues.

The committee could not identify any definitive evidence about the impact regulation would have on the innovation of health IT. Because health IT is a rapidly developing technology and its impact on patient safety is highly dependent on implementation and design, the committee believes policy makers need to be cognizant of not restricting the positive innovation or flexibility needed to improve patient safety. However, legal barriers imposed by contracts between vendors and users may prevent the sharing of safety-related health IT information and hinder the development of a shared learning environment. To encourage innovation and shared learning environments, the committee adopted the following general principles for government oversight:

- Focus on shared learning,
- Maximize transparency,
- Be nonpunitive,

- Identify appropriate levels of accountability, and
- Minimize burden.

The committee considered the various levels of oversight that would be appropriate and focused on areas where private-sector efforts by themselves would not likely result in improved safety. In particular, the committee considered a number of mechanisms to complement the private sector in filling the previously identified knowledge gaps. To achieve safer health care, the committee considers the following actions—when coupled with private-sector efforts—to be the minimum levels of government oversight needed:

- Vendor registration and listing of health IT products;
- Consistent use of quality management principles in the design and use of products;
- Regular public reporting of health IT–related adverse events to encourage transparency; and
- Aggregation, analysis, and investigation of reports of health IT–related adverse events.

The committee categorized health IT–related adverse events as deaths, serious injuries, and unsafe conditions.[4] While deaths and serious injuries are concrete evidence of harm that has already occurred, unsafe conditions can represent the precursors of the events that cause death and serious injuries and are generally greater in volume and provide the proactive opportunity to identify vulnerabilities and mitigate them before any patient is harmed. Analysis of unsafe conditions would produce important information that could potentially have a greater impact on systemically improving patient safety and would enable the adoption of corrective actions that could prevent death or serious injury.

Registration of Vendors and Listing of Products

As a first step toward transparency and improving safety, it is necessary to identify the products being used and to whom any communications or actions about a product need to be directed. As learned from a variety of industries (such as medical devices and pharmaceuticals), vendor registration and listing of products is necessary to hold makers accountable for the safety of their products. Registration and listing can also serve as a resource

---

[4] The committee recognizes that a number of terms are used to describe potential events and conditions unsafe for patients, otherwise known in this section as unsafe conditions. Other terms include close calls, near misses, hazards, and malfunctions that could lead to death or serious injury.

for purchasers to know what products are available in the market when selecting a health IT product. Having a mechanism to accomplish this is important so that when new knowledge about safety or performance arises that is specific to a product and is developed independent of a vendor, other users, and products that could also be vulnerable, can be identified.

The committee believes it is important that vendors of complete EHRs and EHR modules[5] register with a centralized body and continue to list their products. This should eventually include vendors of all health IT products. Seeing that creators of internally developed EHR systems are also considered under the meaningful use program, they should continue to be included as vendors that need to register and list their products.

In determining what organization would be appropriate to register manufacturers and house a list of products, the committee considered FDA and the ONC as the most logical organizations to support these functions. According to the director of FDA's Center for Devices and Radiological Health, FDA has authority to regulate health IT but has not yet exercised it for some types of health IT such as EHRs[6] (Shuren, 2010). FDA currently requires that manufacturers of pharmaceutical drugs and medical devices register with FDA and list their products through a fee-based system. However, pharmaceutical drugs and medical devices are very different from health IT products such as EHRs, health information exchanges, and personal health records.

As part of the meaningful use program, the ONC employed a similar mechanism for EHR vendors to list their products. For health care providers to be able to qualify for EHR incentive payments, they must use a complete EHR or EHR module that meets specific certification criteria established by the ONC. ONC-ATCBs certify specific products based on these criteria and report certified products to the ONC on a weekly basis. The ONC collects and makes this information available to the public; the data are also available to allow purchasers to make more informed decisions about the systems they are interested in purchasing.[7] The ONC therefore already has relationships in place with vendors and would be able to conduct this function without requiring a new mechanism, limiting any confusion that may arise as a result of duplicating an already-existing system.

The committee concludes that the ONC is a better option than FDA

---

[5] The ONC defines a complete EHR as a "technology that has been developed to meet, at a minimum, all applicable certification criteria adopted by the Secretary" and an EHR module as "any service, component, or combination thereof that can meet the requirements of at least one certification criterion adopted by the Secretary" (HHS, 2010).

[6] FDA regulates some types of health IT, for example tools for storing laboratory data, decision support (e.g., prescription dose calculators), and technology related to blood banks (Shuren, 2010).

[7] The certified health IT product list can be found at http://onc-chpl.force.com/ehrcert (accessed April 20, 2011).

and supports continuation of the ONC's efforts to list all products certified for meaningful use in a single database as a first step for ensuring safety.

> Recommendation 5: All health IT vendors should be required to publicly register and list their products with the ONC, initially beginning with EHRs certified for the meaningful use program.

Adopting Quality Systems Toward Safer Health IT

The committee also considered enhancing the mechanisms for health IT vendors to ensure the safety of their products. Quality management principles and processes have been in place in industries such as defense and manufacturing since the early 20th century. These quality management principles and processes were first developed in response to military needs for quality inspection and evolved into a more comprehensive approach of identifying responsibilities for the production staff (American Society for Quality, 2011). These industries' adoption of formal processes to continually improve the effectiveness, efficiency, and overall quality of their systems helped drive their products toward safety and reliability while still supporting innovation.

The same outcome can occur in health IT. Because quality management principles and processes focus on driving performance characteristics at each level to make sure that the product and specifications are in line with the users' needs and expectations, they can help health IT vendors take into account characteristics such as interoperability, usability, and human factors principles as they design and develop safer products.

Examples of Quality Management Principles and Processes

Numerous industries have set standards for quality management principles and processes to help identify, track, and monitor both known and unknown safety hazards. Some examples of quality management principles and processes include the following: the Hazard Analysis Critical Control Point (HACCP) system, FDA Quality System Regulation (QSR), and the International Organization for Standardization (ISO) standards and principles. These examples of quality management principles and processes are designed to afford organizations the flexibility to develop their own processes to best suit their needs as long as these processes meet standard criteria. The examples presented are not meant to be inclusive or to indicate that one process is superior to the other. They are instead meant to illustrate what currently exists in other industries, what could be included in a process to ensure safety and quality with health IT, and how such processes could benefit the health IT industry.

A HACCP system, primarily used by the food industry as a quality system, is a proactive and preventive approach to applying both technical and scientific principles to ensure the reliability, quality, and safety of a product (Dahiya et al., 2009). Prior to implementation of a HACCP system, certain organizational prerequisites and preliminary tasks must be conducted to ensure that the environment supports the production of safe products. These tasks include assembling a team of individuals knowledgeable about the product and the processes involved in creating the product, as well as describing the product, its intended use, and its intended distribution. After these tasks have been completed, the focus can shift to implementing a HACCP system.

HACCP systems comprise seven principles that work together to help identify, prevent, track, and monitor hazards and aid in reducing risks that may occur at specific points in the product life cycle (see Figure 6-1) (Dahiya et al., 2009). Several of these principles can be important for use within the health IT industry, including the following: conducting a hazard analysis, determining critical control points, establishing monitoring procedures, and establishing corrective actions. Conducting a hazard analysis allows unsafe conditions to be identified prior to product completion and implementation in a health care setting. This is a preventive measure that enables vendors to determine critical control points that are then applied to prevent, eliminate, or mitigate the risk. These critical control points are then monitored to determine if they are under control or if a deviation has occurred. Finally, corrective actions are established to help determine the cause of a product deviation and what actions if any were taken to correct the issue. HACCP systems are used in the dairy, meat, and fish and seafood industries and are currently being adapted for use in the pharmaceutical industry.

Another example of quality management principles and processes can be found in FDA's QSR for medical devices, which are also called current good manufacturing practices. A QSR is a set of interrelated or interacting elements organizations use to direct and control how quality policies are implemented and how quality objectives are achieved. FDA's QSR helps ensure medical devices are safe and effective for their intended use by requiring both domestic and foreign device manufacturers to have a quality system that accomplishes the following outcomes: establish various specifications and controls for devices; design devices to meet the specifications of a quality system; manufacture devices based on the principles of a quality system; ensure finished devices meet these specifications; correctly install, check, and service devices; analyze quality data to identify and correct quality problems; and process complaints (FDA, 2009).

Like the HACCP principles, the subsystems under the FDA quality management principles and processes (see Figure 6-2) may be applied to

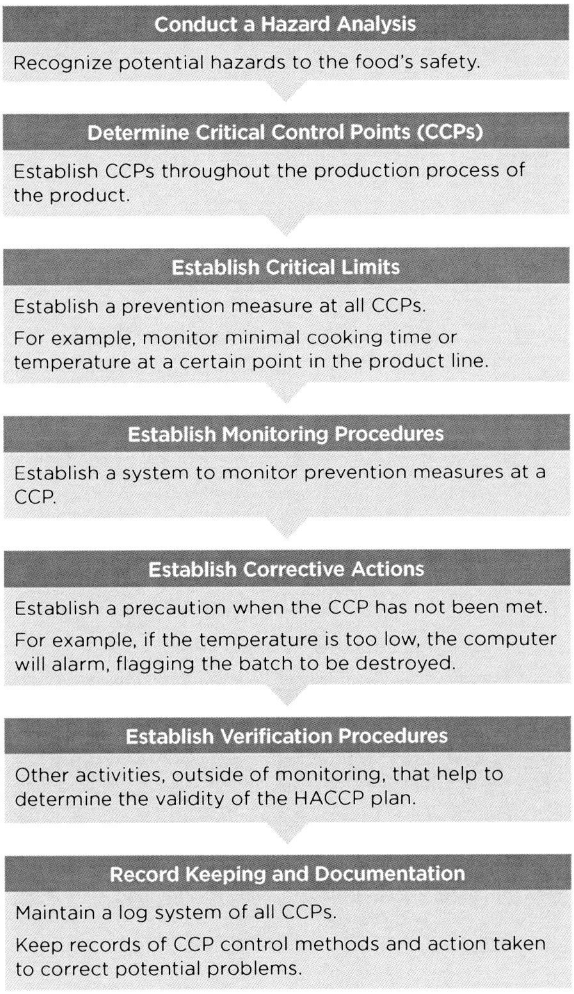

Conduct a Hazard Analysis

Recognize potential hazards to the food's safety.

Determine Critical Control Points (CCPs)

Establish CCPs throughout the production process of the product.

Establish Critical Limits

Establish a prevention measure at all CCPs.

For example, monitor minimal cooking time or temperature at a certain point in the product line.

Establish Monitoring Procedures

Establish a system to monitor prevention measures at a CCP.

Establish Corrective Actions

Establish a precaution when the CCP has not been met.

For example, if the temperature is too low, the computer will alarm, flagging the batch to be destroyed.

Establish Verification Procedures

Other activities, outside of monitoring, that help to determine the validity of the HACCP plan.

Record Keeping and Documentation

Maintain a log system of all CCPs.

Keep records of CCP control methods and action taken to correct potential problems.

FIGURE 6-1
Principles of the HACCP system.

SOURCE: Adapted from Dahiya et al. (2009).

health IT. In particular, the management subsystem and the production and process controls subsystem may be useful in considering what quality management principles apply to health IT. The management subsystem can be useful within health IT because it emphasizes the importance of management's role in making sure quality management principles and pro-

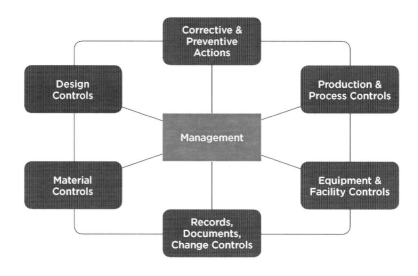

FIGURE 6-2
QMS subsystems.

SOURCE: FDA (2011).

cesses are in place, such as completing quality audits to ensure employee compliance, and making employees aware of known product defects and errors. In addition, the production and process control subsystem allows for changes within product specification, methods, and procedures by allowing revalidation by the vendor to ensure that changes have not altered the intended use and usability of the product. This validation would be done by inspecting, testing, and verifying that the product conforms to its intended use and distribution.

Another proactive technique to characterize hazards, prioritize them for mitigation, and develop mitigation action plans is the Healthcare Failure Modes and Effects Analysis (HFMEA®). This methodology was developed by the National Center for Patient Safety at the U.S. Department of Veterans Affairs (VA) and is an amalgam of HACCP and traditional failure modes and effects analysis. HFMEA has been used for many patient safety–related issues including bar-coding for medication administration (DeRosier et al., 2002).

Another example of quality management principles and processes can be found with ISO, which sets standards for industries around the world. The ISO 9000 series is a quality management process based on eight principles to be used by an organization's senior management as a framework toward improved performance (ISO, 2011). The eight principles are customer focus, leadership, involvement of people, process approach, systems approach management, continual improvement, factual approach to decision making, and mutually beneficial supplier relationships. Generally, these principles are considered to be more comprehensive than other quality management principles and processes, including both HACCP and FDA QSR, because they apply basic quality controls to the whole system, including design and servicing. In addition to quality, ISO also provides guidance in the areas of safety and effectiveness and risk management. Finally, ISO standards have been developed to provide guidance on health informatics to manufacturers interested in producing EHRs as well as supporting interoperability and usability.

Application to Health IT Vendors

The adoption of quality management processes and principles have been demonstrated to improve product safety in other fields; therefore, the committee believes the adoption of quality management principles and processes to be critical to improving the safety of health IT (Chow-Chua et al., 2003; Glasgow et al., 2010, Johansen et al., 2011; VanRooyen et al., 1999). The committee is aware that many vendors already have some type of quality management principles and processes in place. However, not all vendors do, and the level of comprehensiveness of these quality management principles and processes is unknown. An industry standard is needed to ensure comprehensive quality management principles and processes are adopted throughout the health IT industry to provide health care organizations and the general public assurance that health IT products meet a minimum level of safety, reliability, and usability.

To this end, the committee believes adoption of quality management principles and processes should be mandatory for all health IT vendors. Oversight is needed to ensure compliance with these quality management principles and processes once they are in place. The committee considered four entities that could potentially oversee this process: FDA, the ONC, current ONC-ATCBs, and professional societies such as HIMSS.

As discussed earlier, vendors of FDA-regulated industries (e.g., medical devices, food, biologics, drugs) are required to have adopted quality management principles and processes. This risk-based framework is periodically inspected either when a concern is suspected or as part of a schedule and allows vendors to assess regulatory compliance. In addition, FDA has the ability to enforce and take other actions against those vendors who are not compliant with these regulations. Although the QSR provides vendors with flexibility, the committee does not believe the current quality system is the correct process needed for overseeing the health IT industry because it emphasizes regulation of design and labeling. Instead, there may be principles within the QSR that may provide guidance to vendors of health IT.

The committee also considered the ONC's potential role. Although the ONC is not operationally oriented like FDA, it already has relationships with health IT vendors. The ONC could build on the principles of the aforementioned examples and develop a standard baseline set of principles upon which vendors could conform their products and processes. This would create a minimum standard for the industry while also allowing vendors flexibility without fear of regulation.

Another option is for the ONC-ATCBs to require that such processes be adopted as part of their certification criteria for the meaningful use program. Vendors who wish to have their EHR certified for meaningful use are currently working with these certifying bodies, so a relationship already exists. While oversight would fall to these certifying bodies, they could coordinate with the appropriate organization to develop processes that would aid in guiding the development of safer health IT. However, having the responsibility diffused among a number of the ONC-ATCBs may be problematic because of the difficulty of ensuring all organizations hold the vendors to the same level of scrutiny. Furthermore, the committee considers quality management principles and processes to be critical for the safety of health IT products and therefore does not want to limit the adoption of quality management principles and processes to those vendors participating in the meaningful use program.

Finally, the committee discussed the role of professional associations and societies such as HIMSS. Professional associations can help to provide guidance to the industry by setting and adopting current national and international standards, establishing industry recommended practices, and issuing recommendations. Similar to the ONC-ATCB option, professional associations in turn could work with a governmental body like FDA or an organization like ISO to establish guidelines comparable to those in other industries. However, there is concern that HIMSS and other professional associations and societies may not be appropriate because they have a significant amount of industry sponsorship that could jeopardize their ability to serve as neutral parties.

The ONC, FDA, and the ONC-ATCBs are examples of organizations that could all potentially administer this function. In the absence of other information, the Secretary of HHS should determine the most appropriate body.

Recommendation 6: The Secretary of HHS should specify the quality and risk management process requirements that health IT vendors must adopt, with a particular focus on human factors, safety culture, and usability.

In addition to vendors, users of health IT ought to have quality management principles and processes in place to help identify risks. However, the committee could not find any documented evidence to suggest which processes would lead to better outcomes among users.

Regular Reporting of Health IT–Related Deaths, Serious Injuries, or Unsafe Conditions

As discussed previously, to ascertain the volume and types of patient safety risks and to strengthen the market, reports of adverse patient safety events need to be collected. Regular reporting of adverse events is a widely used practice to identify and rectify vulnerabilities that threaten safety. When adverse events are identified, organizations not only learn from their mistakes but can also share the lessons learned with others to prevent future occurrences. As described in Chapter 3, event reporting is critical to promoting safer systems, especially when work-as-designed drifts from work-in-practice. The previously discussed private-sector reporting system for identifying health IT–related adverse events, while critical, only encourages reporting to a certain level. To drive reporting, it needs to be supplemented with a comprehensive reporting system.

Reporting Systems in Other Industries

The experiences of reporting systems both in health care and other industries have shown that it is critical to create an environment that encourages reporting. In the United States, a number of industries have mechanisms to collect reports of adverse events, including aviation, rail, industrial chemicals, nuclear power, and pharmaceuticals. One leading example of a reporting system for close calls is the NASA Aviation Safety Reporting System (ASRS). Under the auspices of ASRS, reports of hazards in which aviation safety may have been compromised are submitted voluntarily (accidents—instances involving actual harm—are not accepted and are referred to other agencies such as the Federal Aviation Administration [FAA] and the National Transportation Safety Board [NTSB]). ASRS compiles the deidentified, verified reports in a publicly accessible database. Once the reports have been deidentified, NASA retains no information that would allow association with the initial reporter; the program has not had a breach in confidentiality in its more than 30-year history. The FAA also makes two other commitments to the aviation community: (a) it does not use ASRS reports against reporting parties in enforcement actions, and (b) it waives fines and penalties under many circumstances for unintentional violations of federal aviation statutes and regulations that are reported to ASRS (NASA, 2011a).

Provision (a) states that information provided by reporting parties will not be used against them, and it addresses the fear that information contained in a report will be used against the reporting party. Provision (b) goes farther in that it offers actual immunity under specified circumstances for safety incidents if a report has been properly filed, regardless of how knowledge of the harm comes to light. (Reporting parties may be found in violation of an aviation regulation, but no punitive actions will be taken under specified circumstances.) Provision (b) thus provides an affirmative incentive for reporting (NASA, 2011b).

Despite the success of ASRS, it is not a comprehensive system. ASRS does not receive reports of actual adverse events and does not have the ability to conduct thorough investigations as to causative factors within the sociotechnical system. Therefore, confidentiality and immunity are only conferred for reports of close calls and not actual harm. Identifying patterns of occurrences is not the same as identifying the underlying causes. This is a critical point because without identification of the underlying causes, it can be difficult if not impossible to formulate a coherent and effective action plan to mitigate the risk to patients.

Reporting Systems in Health Care

Testimony to the U.S. Senate in 2000 noted that "[a]pproaches that focus on punishing individuals instead of changing systems provide strong incentives for people to report only those errors they cannot hide. Thus, a punitive approach shuts off the information that is needed to identify faulty systems and create safer ones. In a punitive system, no one learns from their mistakes" (U.S. Congress, 2000). Reporting systems currently exist in health care to protect patient safety both in other countries and within the United States. Reporting systems have long been in place in countries such as Denmark, the Netherlands, Switzerland, and the United Kingdom. These systems all differ with respect to their design, but some common themes have emerged: reporting ought to be nonpunitive, confidential, independent, evaluated by experts, timely, systems-oriented, and responsive. The term nonpunitive is used here to mean that reports of health IT–related adverse events should be free from punishment or retaliation as a result of reporting. Some systems mandate reports of adverse events and patient safety incidents, while others allow for confidential, voluntary reporting (WHO, 2005).

Within the United States, a few disparate adverse event reporting systems have been developed by groups such as The Joint Commission, the Department of Veterans Affairs (VA), individual states, and more recently at a national level, through the patient safety organizations (PSOs):

- The Joint Commission requires reports of sentinel events[8] to be submitted for health care organizations to receive accreditation. Organizations are expected to conduct their own investigations of sentinel events and submit a report of both the process and results to The Joint Commission for verification. If reports are not up to standard, organizations have the opportunity to fix the reports or their accreditation status may be reviewed (The Joint Commission, 2011).
- The VA developed two complementary nonpunitive reporting systems, the external NASA/VA Patient Safety Reporting System and the internal VA National Center for Patient Safety reporting system. The NASA/VA Patient Safety Reporting System is an external, nonpunitive system modeled after NASA ASRS and accepts reports of close calls and actual adverse events where harm has occurred. Reports are protected from disclosure and no individuals are identified explicitly in these reports or in the subsequent safety investigations. Like its sister system, NASA ASRS, the NASA/VA Patient Safety Reporting System *does not* do comprehensive investigations as to causation or track implementation for countermeasures. It was developed as a safety valve where reporters unwilling to report to the internal VA National Center for Patient Safety reporting system could make their concerns known. The internal, nonpunitive VA National Center for Patient Safety reporting system received more than 1,000 reports for every report received by the NASA/VA Patient Safety Reporting System over a 10-year period (Bagian et al., 2001). The VA National Center for Patient Safety reporting system *does* formulate action plans for reports of events, tracking implementation, effectiveness of interventions, and mechanisms for dissemination, and for this reason is the mechanism that affords the greater potential to improve safety.
- At the state level, 26 states currently require mandatory reporting of adverse events and 1 state has a system in place for voluntary reporting (National Academy for State Health Policy, 2010).
- FDA requires manufacturers of pharmaceutical drugs, therapeutic biologic products, and medical devices to report adverse events to its MedWatch program. The general public and health care providers also are encouraged, although not required, to voluntarily submit reports of adverse events to FDA.
- Clinicians and health care organizations can confidentially report patient safety work product (not just adverse events related to health IT) to the PSOs, which operate under the purview of

---

[8] The Joint Commission defines sentinel event as "an unexpected occurrence involving death or serious physical or psychological injury, or the risk thereof" (The Joint Commission, 2011).

AHRQ.[9] The PSOs are intended to analyze patient safety reports to identify patterns and to propose measures to eliminate patient safety risks and hazards.

Despite the existence of these and other systems and many calls for change, reports of adverse events in the United States currently are not collected in a comprehensive manner. Furthermore, learning from these systems is limited because a multitude of different data is collected by each system, hampering any attempt to aggregate data between reporting systems. It is also the case that users are being asked to notify multiple reporting systems; the burden of multiple reporting systems can potentially discourage reporting. As previously discussed, the Common Formats effort is under way to streamline the types of data being collected, which serves as a first step to collecting similar data across reporting systems. It must be emphasized, however, that these reporting systems are not intended or capable of furnishing accurate counts or prevalence and incidence data. Instead, their purpose is to identify vulnerabilities and hazards that can then be prioritized for the institution of corrective actions to mitigate the identified risks.

The committee believes systems that encourage both vendors and users to report health IT–related adverse events are needed to improve the safety of patient care. Evaluations of reporting systems examined by the committee indicate that well-designed voluntary reporting can improve safety (Leape, 2002) in an environment that encourages reporting. To create an environment that encourages reporting, reporters' identities need to be kept confidential; it is important to note that protections of privilege and confidentiality generally refer to reports by users and not manufacturers of products. In addition, if the reports do not result in action or if actions that are taken are not provided as feedback to the reporters, the sustainability of the reporting system can be impacted negatively. Perhaps more important is that reports for the purpose of learning have to be separate from the purpose of addressing accountability. An environment that does not allow reporting parties to be punished as a result of reporting is critical for the success of voluntary reporting systems.

---

[9] As of August 2011, 81 PSOs were listed (AHRQ, 2011b). These organizations receive reports of events from providers, provide feedback and recommendations to the reporting providers, and deidentify reports and send the data to AHRQ for incorporation into a network of patient safety databases. However, it is important that data received by the PSOs are not deidentified and scrubbed of all data that would make data unuseful for drawing trends, such as what technology, product, and module number are being used.

Reporting of Health IT–Related Adverse Events

A subset of adverse events can be identified as being related to health IT. Health IT–related events can occur in every setting and level of health care but currently are not required to be reported. As a result, shared knowledge of such events is incomplete and any effort to understand and prevent such events from occurring in the future is far from optimal. The committee believes it is in the best interest of the public for deidentified, verified health IT–related adverse events to be released transparently to the public for the purpose of shared learning, and the responsibility for identifying and reporting events lies with both vendors and users of health IT. Although reporting could also be done by patients and the general public, the committee believes vendors and users are the only actors that should be responsible formally for reporting adverse events and that they have distinct roles in this regard. Coupled with the suggested private-sector system for reporting, a comprehensive public–private system that supports an environment for reporting can be created.

Reports of health IT–related death, serious injury, and unsafe conditions should be collected. Those events falling into the unsafe conditions category may be especially difficult to detect, for example, events that arise as a result of usability issues that do not result in immediate patient harm. Based on the experiences from the VA National Center for Patient Safety reporting system and others, the committee concludes reporting systems should not receive submissions of intentionally unsafe acts;[10] instead, intentionally unsafe acts ought to be relayed to the health care organizations themselves to follow regular legal channels. In this way, the goal of the reporting system remains focused on learning and not accountability.

Reports by Vendors

For health IT–related adverse events, the onus of reporting does not fall solely on users. The committee believes all vendors should collect and act on reports of adverse events. Some vendors collect, review, and act on reports of adverse events from both internal and external sources in a variety of ways (e.g., issue alerts to health care providers who may be affected) (IOM, 2011). Vendors are not required to report adverse events if their products are not regulated by FDA currently, although some health IT vendors voluntarily report to the FDA MedWatch Safety Information and Adverse Event Reporting Program (IOM, 2011). However, because vendors do not perform these tasks in a consistent way or share experi-

---

[10] Intentionally unsafe acts in this context can be defined as "events that result from a criminal act, a purposefully unsafe act, or an act related to alcohol or substance abuse or patient abuse" (Veterans Affairs National Center for Patient Safety, 2011).

ences, instances of harm and any lessons learned from them are not shared systematically.

The committee concludes that reporting of deaths, serious injuries, or unsafe conditions should be mandatory for vendors and that an entity be given the authority to act on these reports. The ability to take action would allow imminent threats to safety to be addressed immediately and could provide valuable information for future activities and development work. These reports should be collected by an entity for the purpose of learning and therefore should not be used for punitive purposes. A mandate entails expectations that vendors will report adverse events and that some sort of penalty would result for failing to report events.

To create a program of mandatory reporting, direction will need to come from a federal entity with adequate expertise, capacity, and authority to act. This entity could either collect the reports itself or could coordinate with and delegate to the private sector to the extent possible. Precedence for delegation exists, such as the delegation of certification of EHRs by the ONC to a number of the ONC-ATCBs. FDA currently has the capability to require mandatory reporting if it exercised its discretion in regulating EHRs and it has an existing infrastructure for reporting adverse events, but, as discussed in previous sections, the committee does not believe FDA currently has the capacity to do so unless given adequate resources. An authority needs to be designated by the Secretary of HHS to require and act on reports of health IT–related adverse events, and be provided with resources to do so.

Reports by Users

Given the variability in implementing health IT, users of health IT—primarily clinicians as the end users and provider organizations—should be encouraged to report adverse events voluntarily, which should be non-punitive. One mechanism to encourage reporting is to have mechanisms available to easily report hazards and harms (e.g., a button embedded in an EHR screen that allows for one-click reporting). As stated earlier, self-reports are intended to identify vulnerabilities and hazards; they cannot be considered to represent incidence and prevalence of adverse events accurately or prove causation. This is illustrated by a recent study that found adverse events occur in 33 percent of hospital admissions but that local hospital reporting systems identified only 1 percent of those events (Classen et al., 2011), signaling underreporting in voluntary systems. Additionally, the numerous, uncoordinated reporting efforts can result in confusion as to what information ought to be reported, to what system, and in what format. A more streamlined system for reporting is needed so that people are not being asked to relay similar data about the same event multiple times. The committee believes the complexity and frequency of reporting would make mandatory reporting for users infeasible. A reporting system that collects the same information precisely defining the components of a health IT–related adverse event is needed, such as the Common Formats.

The committee therefore concludes that reports by users should remain voluntary and that the identities of reporters should not be discoverable under any circumstance. User-reported health IT–related adverse events should be collected by a central repository and also be sent to the appropriate vendor. In this way, the vendor can also be notified of the event and take precautions and warn other users that may be at risk for an adverse event.

FDA, NASA, AHRQ, states, and others are all able to collect users' reports of health IT–related adverse events. As discussed earlier, the complexity of health IT differs so greatly from FDA's current portfolio that the committee believes FDA would have to institute approaches that are different from their current approach were they to oversee a health IT–related adverse event reporting program for users. NASA has operated ASRS and patient safety reporting systems and has a strong history in keeping reports confidential, but it is not clear that it is positioned to take on a responsibility of this magnitude. The PSO program is just beginning to take shape and is yet to be proven as a comprehensive network for report collection, but it boasts strong confidentiality protections and a widespread presence, and it is tied to a national patient safety database network. Many states have their own reporting requirements, but promoting a disjointed system of reporting limits the ability for systematic collection of reports across the country. The protections offered in the PSO program lead the committee to believe that the PSO program may be the best option for collecting reports from users, but further evidence will need to be collected to validate the success of this approach for user reporting of health IT issues.

> Recommendation 7: The Secretary of HHS should establish a mechanism for both vendors and users to report health IT–related deaths, serious injuries, or unsafe conditions.
>   a. Reporting of health IT–related adverse events should be mandatory for vendors.
>   b. Reporting of health IT–related adverse events by users should be voluntary, confidential, and nonpunitive.
>   c. Efforts to encourage reporting should be developed, such as removing the perceptual, cultural, contractual, legal, and logistical barriers to reporting.

Perceptual, Cultural, and Logistical Barriers to Reporting

As mentioned earlier, multiple barriers prevent sharing and reporting of adverse events. In addition to the previously discussed legal issues, there are also perceptual, cultural, and logistical barriers to reporting. These barriers inhibit not only users' abilities to report to the government, but also sharing of health IT–related adverse events with vendors, other users, and consumer groups. To have an adequate system of reporting and shared learning, each of these barriers needs to be addressed. Indeed, even the best-designed health IT product will inevitably have some content that might contribute to adverse events. Once this is recognized by both providers and manufacturers, disclosure of events can be viewed as the beginning of a shared effort to recognize, fix, and improve patient safety issues.

Clinicians may also be faced with cultural barriers within their own organization. Although reporting of all adverse events has been encouraged for many years, providers may be more reluctant to report those related to health IT because acquiring a health IT product is an expensive, lengthy, and time-consuming investment. After spending a lot of time and resources to adopt health IT, health care organizations may be reluctant to acknowledge that the product may be flawed. Therefore, in the eyes of management, reporting can be viewed as blaming decision makers for implementing a flawed system. This may lead to a culture where health professionals fear that reporting may be viewed as opposing management decisions. These organizations need to recognize that, no matter how well planned the selection and integration of health IT are, problems can arise. Organizational leadership needs to not only encourage reporting, but also view it as a necessary step to improve a complex system that will inevitably have problems.

The logistics of reporting may also be a barrier to reporting. Many health IT–related adverse events occur during treatment, when finding ways to continue care is a higher priority than reporting the problem. Afterward, clinicians may have little time to submit a report of the event or may not remember the full details of the event. Vendors need to create an easy system where clinicians can quickly and easily report. Also, clinicians may be less motivated to report when they do not believe vendors will use the report to change their systems. Vendors and users need to communicate more effectively by providing feedback to each other and making it known that reporting can lead to changes. Each organization and vendor will have its own unique set of barriers; however, the committee believes the potential benefits are worth the burden reporting would impose on vendors and users.

Aggregating, Analyzing, and Investigating
Reports of Health IT–Related Adverse Events

The previous sections and recommendations detail a comprehensive plan that creates an environment to understand the risks and encourage change. This next section focuses on actions that can be taken in response to reports of health IT–related incidents to inform and prevent future events and unsafe conditions from occurring.

Reports of patient safety incidents are critical but are only one part of a larger solution to maximize the safety of health IT–assisted care. As discussed above, reports from vendors, users, or patients alone are generally not complete or detailed enough to understand fully the events leading to an incident and/or to develop solutions that would avert future problems. What is reported is often not completely reflective of what actually occurred.

As illustrated by the creation of the NTSB and the Nuclear Regulatory Commission (NRC) to oversee safety in high-reliability industries such as transportation and nuclear energy, the committee notes that the power to improve safety lies not only with requiring reports of safety incidents, but also with the ability to act on and learn from reports.

Thus, in addition to reporting, two additional activities are needed: (1) aggregating and analyzing data from reports and (2) investigating the circumstances and environment associated with safety incidents to try to identify the conditions that contribute to those incidents. Through these processes, lessons learned can be developed and disseminated so that similar incidents will be less likely to occur in the future. To maximize the effectiveness of reports, the collection, aggregation and analysis, and investigation of reports should be coupled as closely as possible.

Aggregation of reports of health IT–related adverse events—reports of deaths, serious injury, or unsafe conditions—should be conducted to identify patterns. Analyses of these reports can lead to identification of specific patient safety risks, potentially particular to a specific vendor or product. Such examination and additional investigation, where indicated, can lead to development of recommended practices or lessons learned and, potentially, prevent harm to patients.

Reports of adverse events can generate material that supports learning, but analysis is needed to obtain full value from such material. Although retrospective, an investigative function that comprehensively examines the conditions that contribute to health IT–related adverse events is critical so that concrete actions can then be taken proactively to reduce harm.

A Reporting System for Learning and Improving Patient Safety

On their own, vendors and users generally do not have the broad expertise needed to conduct investigations as envisioned by the committee. Vendors and users also may not be impartial arbiters of why an adverse event occurred. As a result, external methods are needed to conduct rigorous investigations of health IT–related adverse events.

Reports could be aggregated and analyzed by multiple entities, such as the PSOs, but trends in data may not be as easily identified if spread out among the more than 80 PSOs because of the smaller number of reports each organization would receive. Additionally, standards of analysis may not be used in the same way across multiple entities, calling into question the reliability of the analyses conducted. Ideally, as depicted in Figure 6-3, reports of health IT–related adverse events or unsafe conditions from both users and vendors would be aggregated and analyzed by a single entity that would identify reports for immediate investigation.

Reports to this entity would have to include identifiable data to allow for investigators to follow up in the event the reported incident requires investigation, but, as discussed previously, full confidentiality protections must be applied to the reports. Reports would need to be received in an identifiable manner from the PSOs or another collecting agency and with enough information to investigate (e.g., specific vendor, model number).

The entity would have the discretion to investigate two categories of reports: (1) novel reports that result in death or serious injury and (2) trends of reports of unsafe conditions (e.g., multiple health care organizations find that a specific pharmacy system accepts only 100 characters of a particular EHR's notes section that allows 125 characters, resulting in the incorrect filling of orders). Prioritization among the reports would be determined on a risk-based hazard analysis. Cases resulting in death or serious injury should be investigated immediately. Reports should be kept confidential and nonpunitive for the purposes of learning. Reports of unsafe conditions should be analyzed and monitored continually and investigated using a risk-based hazard analysis. Which reports to investigate ought to be determined by the explicit risk-based prioritization system that the investigatory entity employs. Reports by vendors should already contain identifiable data.

In keeping with the principle of transparency, reports and results of investigations should be made public. Public release of results of investigations could build off the NTSB process, which separates facts discovered by the investigators from opinions and conclusions drawn by the investigators. A feedback loop from the investigatory body back to both the vendors and users is essential to allow groups to rectify any systemic issues that were found to introduce risk into their systems.

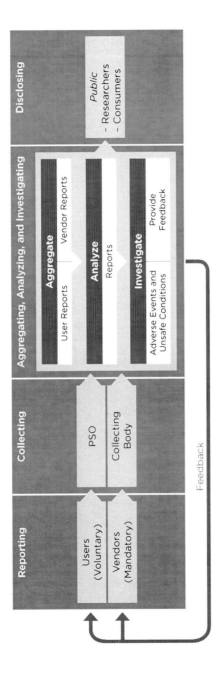

FIGURE 6-3
Reporting system for learning and improving patient safety.

Potential Actors

It is the intent of the committee to build on the current patient safety environment and to maximize the potential for all stakeholders to have a part in ensuring patient safety. However, for the reasons mentioned above, the current system does not adequately address the significant needs of a comprehensive process to learn from health IT–related patient safety risks. A unique knowledge base is needed to understand thoroughly and diagnose ways to improve the interface between health care delivery and health IT, which, as discussed in Chapter 3, is extraordinarily complex and requires the understanding of a large number of sociotechnical domains.

The committee considered a variety of alternatives to objectively analyze reports of unsafe events as well as conduct investigations into health IT–related adverse events in the way the committee envisions. The alternatives considered include FDA, AHRQ, the CMS, the ONC, and entities in the private sector.

- FDA is largely an oversight entity. Adding investigative responsibilities of the nature envisioned by the committee would be at odds with its oversight functions. Additionally, FDA lacks the resources in terms of capacity and expertise, limiting its ability to act in this area.
- AHRQ primarily supports research and technical assistance activities regarding quality and safety. It is not an oversight or investigative agency. AHRQ is also not an active implementer and is not operationally oriented. For AHRQ to take on the functions envisioned by the committee would require a complete change in the agency's charge and internal expertise.
- The CMS is an administrative agency that has demonstrated its leverage with users of health IT through the development of the EHR incentive program and conditions of participation. These programs, while important, contain punitive elements and are inappropriate for completing the aggregative, analytic, and investigative functions described above. The CMS also has little internal expertise relating to clinical workflow and use of technology to support cognition and therefore does not have the infrastructure needed to support these tasks. Additionally, while the CMS could potentially serve in this role, the CMS's authority focuses on providers associated with Medicare and Medicaid and is not as expansive as the committee believes is needed.
- The ONC coordinates health IT efforts and influences the development of policy related to health IT but has no formal authority in this area; it is not an operating division of HHS. It is not clear to

the committee that the ONC has the clinical and operations expertise to conduct investigations of health IT–related adverse events.

- Private-sector organizations such as The Joint Commission, the NCQA, and the NQF play an important role in ensuring safety. However, these organizations are mostly dependent on short-term funding streams, often seeking "soft money" to sustain specific projects and programs. As a result, programmatic content may be shaped in part by funders. Moreover, these groups—even working in collaboration with one another—may not have the far-reaching influences of a federal entity and do not have the mandate or breadth to be able to conduct such investigations at a national level. These groups also do not possess the expertise and ability to properly investigate these issues.

Investigating patient safety incidents related to health IT does not match the internal expertise of any existing entity. Given the status quo, the committee concludes that no existing entity has the necessary attributes to perform the crucial function of investigating health IT–related patient safety incidents as envisioned by the committee. The needed functions are under the jurisdiction of multiple federal agencies, and efforts are uncoordinated and are not as comprehensive as a safety-oriented system ought to be. A multiagency structure could be envisioned, but as discussed previously, oversight and investigative functions should not be housed in the same entity. The committee concludes the envisioned necessary functions cannot be realized solely through current structures, and a new entity is needed that can pull together the following desired goals in an integrated fashion in a way current alternatives cannot achieve:

- A comprehensive system for identifying and investigating deaths, injuries, and unsafe conditions has to be separated explicitly from oversight functions.
- Broad categories of expertise are required to investigate an adverse event fully.
- Vendors and users need to be held accountable publicly for patient deaths, injuries, and potentially unsafe conditions.
- A streamlined approach is needed to reduce wasteful duplication and inconsistencies.
- Lessons from these investigations need to be shared broadly from a respected source so that future adverse events can be averted.

To truly improve patient safety, a new approach is needed. The committee believed that the experiences of other industries such as transportation and nuclear energy in creating the NTSB and the NRC were instructive, and concluded that the development of an independent, federal entity was best suited to performing the needed above-described analytic and investigative functions for health IT–related adverse events in a transparent, nonpunitive manner.

The committee envisions an entity that would be similar in structure to the NTSB or the NRC, which are both independent federal agencies created by and reporting directly to Congress. Among other responsibilities, these entities conduct investigations, for the purpose of ensuring safety. The NTSB is a nonregulatory agency that does not establish fault or liability in the legal sense but investigates incidents. The NRC is a regulatory body that has the ability to issue fines and fees. The committee considered both agencies and concluded the NTSB to be most similar to the needs of health IT–assisted care.

An independent, federal entity analogous in form and function to the NTSB is needed. This entity would not have enforcement power and would be nonpunitive. Instead, it would have the authority to conduct investigations and, upon their completion, make recommendations. The NTSB makes nonbinding recommendations to the Secretary of the Department of Transportation, who then must state within 90 days whether the department intends to perform the recommended procedures in total, carry the recommendations out in part, or refuse to adopt the recommendation. In this case, an entity would make similar recommendations to the Secretary of HHS. Although delivering nonbinding recommendations can be described by some as a flaw, the committee believes that the flexibility it provides is a strength, allowing for the health care organizations, vendors, and external experts to determine the best course forward collectively. If requested by the Secretary, the entity could also perform other functions, such as coordinating with existing bodies, both public and private, as appropriate. Investigations could involve representatives from all impacted parties, including vendors and users involved in the incident, as well as experts in the various sociotechnical dimensions of health IT safety. The committee believes that an independent, federal entity is the best option to provide a platform to support shared learning at a national level. The entity would have the following functions:

- Aggregate reports of health IT–related adverse events from at least vendors and users;
- Analyze the aggregated reports to identify patterns;
- Investigate reports of health IT–related patient deaths or serious injury;
- Investigate trends of reports of unsafe conditions;
- Recommend corrective actions to the Secretary of Health and Human Services;

- Provide feedback to vendors and users following investigations; and
- Disclose results of the investigations to the public, including researchers and consumers.

Recommendation 8: The Secretary of HHS should recommend that Congress establish an independent federal entity for investigating patient safety deaths, serious injuries, or potentially unsafe conditions associated with health IT. This entity should also monitor and analyze data and publicly report results of these activities.

It is also important to recognize that the line between health IT–related adverse events and other adverse events will likely become increasingly blurry. Multiple factors contribute to unsafe conditions and adverse events, making it potentially difficult to differentiate between health IT–related or other factors until an investigation has been conducted. If a broader system for all adverse events is created, the spirit of the committee's recommendations should be recognized and considered.

NEXT STEPS

Patients must be kept safe in the midst of the current large-scale rollout of health IT. While it is clear to the committee that the market has failed to keep patients safe with respect to health IT, the committee believes transparency is the key to improving safety. To truly address health IT safety, many actions will be needed to correct the market; ways to improve flow of communication and correct the market have to be created carefully. When combined, removing contractual restrictions, establishing public reporting, and having a system in place for independent investigations can be a powerful force for improving patient safety.

Achieving transparency, safer health IT products, and safer use of health IT will require the cooperation of all stakeholders. Without more information about the magnitude and types of harm, the committee concluded that other mechanisms were necessary to understand how to best approach health IT safety.

The committee believes the current state of safety and health IT is not acceptable; specific actions are required to improve the safety of health IT. The first eight recommendations are intended to create conditions and incentives to encourage substantial industry-driven change without formal regulation. However, because the private sector to date has not taken substantive action on its own, the committee believes a follow-up recommendation is needed to regulate health IT formally if the actions recommended to the private and public sectors are not effective.[11] If the first eight recommendations are determined by the Secretary of HHS to be not effective, the Secretary should direct FDA to exercise all authorities to regulate health IT.

The committee was of mixed opinion on how FDA regulation would impact the pace of innovation but identified several areas of concern regarding immediate FDA regulation. The current FDA framework is oriented toward conventional, out-of-the-box, turnkey devices. However, health IT has multiple different characteristics, suggesting that a more flexible regulatory framework will be needed in this area to achieve the goals of product quality and safety without unduly constraining market innovation. For example, as a software-based product, health IT has a very different product life cycle than conventional technologies. These products exhibit great diversity in features, functions, and scope of intended and actual use, which tend to evolve over the life of the product. Taking a phased, risk-based approach can help address this concern. FDA has chosen to not exercise regulatory authority as discussed previously, and controversy exists over whether some health IT products such as EHRs should be considered medical devices. If the Secretary deems it necessary to regulate EHRs and other health IT products not currently regulated by FDA, clear determinations will need to be made about whether all health IT products classify as medical devices for the purposes of regulation. The committee also believes that if FDA regulation is deemed necessary, FDA will need to commit sufficient resources and add capacity and expertise to be effective.

The ONC and the Secretary should examine progress critically toward achieving safety and, if needed, determine when to move to the next stage. HHS should report annually to Congress and the public on the progress of efforts to improve the safety of health IT beginning 12 months from the release of this report. In these reports, the Secretary should make clear why she does or does not believe further oversight actions are needed. In parallel, the Secretary should ask FDA to begin planning the framework needed for potential regulation consistent with Recommendations 1 through 8 so that, if she deems FDA regulation to be necessary, the agency will be ready to act, allowing for the protection of patient safety without further delay. FDA will need to coordinate these efforts with the actors identified in Recommendations 1 through 8, including AHRQ and the ONC, among others. In addition, the Secretary will also need to devise new strategies to stimulate the private sector to meet its responsibility of ensuring patient safety. The committee recognizes that not all of its recommendations can be acted on by the Secretary alone and that some will require congressional action.

---

[11] One member disagrees with the committee and would immediately regulate health IT as a Class III medical device, as outlined in Appendix E.

Recommendation 9a: The Secretary of HHS should monitor and publicly report on the progress of health IT safety annually beginning in 2012. If progress toward safety and reliability is not sufficient as determined by the Secretary, the Secretary should direct FDA to exercise all available authorities to regulate EHRs, health information exchanges, and PHRs.

Recommendation 9b: The Secretary should immediately direct FDA to begin developing the necessary framework for regulation. Such a framework should be in place if and when the Secretary decides the state of health IT safety requires FDA regulation as stipulated in Recommendation 9a above.

CONCLUSION

Today the nation is just scaling up with EHRs, and, as a result, the health IT environment is both very dynamic and also stressed. Patient safety is too important to ignore, but clear routes to solid policies that will improve performance are still wanting. Because of the lack of concrete evidence about how to best improve patient safety, the private and public sectors should work together to take the first steps toward identifying the data and building an evidence base for improving health IT–related patient safety. Lessons should be learned from other industries focusing on safety. Although it is important to recognize that none of those reporting systems is perfect, a critical lesson to be learned from these experiences is that safety demands systems of continual learning.

Health IT is a quickly changing field, particularly with respect to outpatient services, and products are being developed continually for the improvement of patient outcomes and more effective care delivery. The functions and types of health IT–related adverse events requiring analysis and investigation will change over time. To this end, the approaches identified in this report should be monitored continually and revised as needed. The identified actor or set of actors should be given the flexibility and latitude to amend its charge as appropriate.

Creating an infrastructure that supports shared learning about and improving the safety of health IT is needed to achieve better health care. Proactive measures have to be taken to ensure health IT products are developed and implemented with safety as a primary focus through the development of industry-wide measures, standards, and criteria for safety. Surveillance mechanisms will be available to identify, capture, and investigate adverse events to improve the safety of health IT continually. Transparency and cooperation between the private and public sectors is the key to creating the necessary infrastructure to build safer systems that will lead to better care for all Americans.

REFERENCES

AHRQ (Agency for Healthcare Research and Quality). 2011a. *Common formats.* http://www. pso.ahrq.gov/formats/commonfmt.htm (accessed May 8, 2011).

AHRQ. 2011b. *Georgraphic directory of listed patient safety organizations.* http://www.pso. ahrq.gov/listing/geolist.htm (accessed August 9, 2011).

American Society for Quality. 2011. *The history of quality—overview.* http://asq.org/learn-about-quality/history-of-quality/overview/overview.html (accessed June 17, 2011).

Bagian, J. P., C. Lee, J. Gosbee, J. DeRosier, E. Stalhandske, N. Eldridge, R. Williams, and M. Burkhardt. 2001. Developing and deploying a patient safety program in a large health care delivery system: You can't fix what you don't know about. *Joint Commission Journal on Quality Improvement* 27(10):522-532.

Chow-Chua, C., M. Goh, and T. B. Wan. 2003. Does ISO 9000 certification improve business performance. *International Journal of Quality & Reliability Management* 20(8):936-953.

Classen, D. C., and D. W. Bates. 2011. Finding the meaning in meaningful use. *New England Journal of Medicine* 365(9):855-858.

Classen, D. C., R. Resar, F. Griffin, F. Federico, T. Frankel, N. Kimmel, J. C. Whittington, A. Frankel, A. Seger, and B. C. James. 2011. "Global trigger tool" shows that adverse events in hospitals may be ten times greater than previously measured. *Health Affairs* 30(4):581-589.

Cohen, L. 1979. Innovation and atomic energy: Nuclear power regulation, 1966-present. *Law and Contemporary Problems* 43(1):67-97.

Cullen, D. J., D. W. Bates, S. D. Small, J. B. Cooper, A. R. Nemeskal, and L. L. Leape. 1995. The incident reporting system does not detect adverse drug events: A problem for quality improvement. *Joint Commission Journal on Quality Improvement* 21(10):541-548.

Dahiya, S., R. K. Khar, and A. Chhikara. 2009. Opportunities, challenges and benefits of using HACCP as a quality risk management tool in the pharmaceutical industry. *Quality Assurance Journal* 12(2):95-104.

DeRosier, J., E. Stalhandske, J. P. Bagian, and T. Nudell. 2002. Using health care failure mode and effect analysis: The VA National Center for Patient Safety's prospective risk analysis system. *Joint Commission Journal on Quality Improvement* 28(5):248-267, 209.

FDA (Food and Drug Administration). 2009. *The quality system regulation.* http://www. fda.gov/MedicalDevices/DeviceRegulationandGuidance/PostmarketRequirements/ QualitySystemsRegulations/MedicalDeviceQualitySystemsManual/ucm122391.htm (accessed June 1, 2011).

Gardner, R. M., J. M. Overhage, E. B. Steen, B. S. Munger, J. H. Holmes, J. J. Williamson, D. E. Detmer, and the AMIA Board of Directors. 2009. Core content for the subspecialty of clinical informatics. *Journal of the American Medical Informatics Association* 16(2):153-157.

Gastineau, D. A. 2004. Will regulation be the death of cell therapy in the United States? *Bone Marrow Transplant* 33(8):777-780.

Glasgow, J., J Scott-Caziewell, and P. Kaboli. 2010. Guiding inpatient quality improvement: A systematic review of lean and six sigma. *Joint Commission Journal on Quality and Patient Safety* 36(12):531-532.

Goodman, K. W., E. S. Berner, M. A. Dente, B. Kaplan, R. Koppel, D. Rucker, D. Z. Sands, P. Winkelstein, and the AMIA Board of Directors. 2011. Challenges in ethics, safety, best practices, and oversight regarding HIT vendors, their customers, and patients: A report of an AMIA special task force. *Journal of the American Medical Informatics Association* 18(1):77-81.

Grabowski, H. G., and J. M. Vernon. 1977. Consumer protection regulation in ethical drugs. *American Economic Review* 67(1):359-364.

Hauptman, O., and E. B. Roberts. 1987. FDA regulation of product risk and its impact upon young biomedical firms. *Journal of Product Innovation Management* 4(2):138-148.

HHS (Department of Health and Human Services). 2010. Health information technology: Initial set of standards, implementation, specifications, and certification criteria for electronic health record technology; final rule. *Federal Register* 75(144):44590-44654.

IOM (Institute of Medicine). 2011 (unpublished). *Vendor responses—summary.* Washington, DC: IOM.

ISO (International Organization for Standardization). 2011. *Quality management principles.* http://www.iso.org/iso/iso_catalogue/management_and_leadership_standards/quality_management/qmp.htm (accessed May 26, 2011).

Johansen, I., M. Bruun-Rasmussen, K. Bourquard, E. Poiseau, M. Zoric, C. Parisot, and M. Onken. 2011. *A quality management system for interoperability testing.* Paper presented at 23rd International Conference of the European Federation for Medical Informatics, Oslo, Norway, August 28, 2011, to August 31, 2011.

The Joint Commission. 2011. *Sentinel events.* Chicago: The Joint Commission.

Kim, D. U. 2002. The quest for quality blood banking program in the new millennium the American way. *International Journal of Hematology* 76(Suppl 2):258-262.

Laflamme, F. M., W. E. Pietraszek, and N. V. Rajadhyax. 2010. Reforming hospitals with IT investment. *McKinsey Quarterly* 20:27-33.

Leape, L. L. 2002. Reporting of adverse events. *New England Journal of Medicine* 347(20):1633-1638.

Marcus, A. A. 1988. Implementing induced innovations: A comparison of rule-bound and autonomous approaches. *Academy of Management Journal* 31(2):235-256.

NASA (National Aeronautics and Space Administration). 2011a. *Confidentiality and incentives to report.* http://asrs.arc.nasa.gov/overview/confidentiality.html (accessed April 18, 2011).

NASA. 2011b. *Immunity policy.* http://asrs.arc.nasa.gov/overview/immunity.html (accessed April 18, 2011).

National Academy for State Health Policy. 2010. *Patient safety toolbox.* http://www.nashp.org/pst-welcome (accessed June 24, 2011).

NIST (National Institute of Standards and Technology). 2006. *Guide to integrating forensic techniques into incident response.* Gaithersburg, MD: NIST.

NIST. 2010. *Computerized common industry format template for electronic health record usability testing.* Gaithersburg, MD: NIST.

NQF (National Quality Forum). 2011. *NQF: Governance and leadership.* http://qualityforum.org/About_NQF/Governance_and_Leadership.aspx (accessed June 24, 2011).

ONC (Office of the National Coordinator for Health Information Technology). 2011. *Health IT workforce development program facts at a glance.* http://healthit.hhs.gov/portal/server.pt?open=512&objID=1432&mode=2 (accessed June 24, 2011).

Quality and Safety Education for Nurses. 2011. *Quality and safety competencies.* http://www.qsen.org/competencies.php (accessed July 19, 2011).

Schneider, P. 1996. FDA & clinical software vendors: A line in the sand? *Healthcare Informatics* 13(6):100-102, 104, 106.

Shuren, J. 2010. Statement to IOM Committee on Patient Safety and Health Information Technology. Statement read at the Workshop of the IOM Committee on Patient Safety and Health Information Technology, Washington, DC.

Sittig, D. F., and D. C. Classen. 2010. Safe electronic health record use requires a comprehensive monitoring and evaluation framework. *Journal of the American Medical Association* 303(5):450-451.

Sittig, D. F., and H. Singh. 2009. Eight rights of safe electronic health record use. *Journal of the American Medical Association* 302(10):1111-1113.

U.S. Congress, Senate Subcommittee on Labor, Health and Human Services, and Education. 2000. *Testimony of Leape, L.*

VanRooyen, M. J., J. G. Grabowski, A. J. Ghidorzi, C. Dey, and G. R. Strange. 1999. The perceived effectiveness of total quality management as a tool for quality improvement in emergency medicine. *Academic Emergency Medicine* 6(8):811-816.

Veterans Affairs National Center for Patient Safety. 2011. *FAQ: How do you define an intentional unsafe act?* http://www.patientsafety.gov/FAQ.html (accessed August 9, 2011).

Walshe, K., and S. M. Shortell. 2004. Social regulation of healthcare organizations in the United States: Developing a framework for evaluation. *Health Services Management Research* 17(2):79-99.

Weeda, D. F., and N. F. O'Flaherty. 1998. Food and Drug Administration regulation of blood bank software: The new regulatory landscape for blood establishments and their vendors. *Transfusion* 38(1):86-89.

WHO (World Health Organization). 2005. *WHO draft guidelines for adverse event reporting and learning systems: From information to action.* Geneva: World Health Organization Press.

7

Future Research for Care Transformation

This chapter focuses on areas of future research that can, in the long term, lead to care transformation and development of safer health IT. The literature shows that with well-designed software and appropriate staff training, health IT can have a positive effect on safety; outside of those conditions, health IT can negatively impact safety. However, the literature is far from complete. A research agenda is needed to help improve patient safety via information technology. The committee discovered a number of research gaps during its information gathering and identified four broad areas: safe design and development of technologies, safe implementation and use of technologies, considerations for researchers, and policy issues. Research is needed to continue to build the evidence to determine how to most effectively and safely adopt health IT. A greater body of conclusive research is needed to fully describe the potential of health IT for ensuring patient safety. This discussion is a starting point and not a comprehensive list.

DESIGN AND DEVELOPMENT OF TECHNOLOGIES

Patient safety depends on the sound design and development of health IT. However, the optimal design or development is unknown and may indeed be impossible to determine. In light of this, research is needed to identify characteristics of safe systems. Some properties of health IT integral to patient safety require further research, including usability, interoperability, understanding the complexity of health care delivery, and the balance between standardization and customization.

Usability is one characteristic of health IT design and development requiring further research. Maximizing usability will ensure clinicians' needs are taken into account in the design of the relevant human–computer interactions. A variety of industry standards may apply to health IT but compliance with standards serves only as a weak screen for design deficiencies. Although general principles of usability are well described and some work around usability is currently under way in health IT, additional research is needed specifically about its impact on patient safety.

Another characteristic of design and development important to safety is interoperability. Interoperability can allow data to be shared readily, for example, between an electronic health record (EHR) and a pharmacy system without loss of semantic content. Interoperability will require harmonization of standards, such as how data can best be formatted and stored. Consistent rules governing transmission of data and use of common terminologies are being developed through health information exchanges; their success will need further inquiry.

Research is needed on interfaces to support the fact that medical care requires the cooperation of multiple health professionals in multiple institutions. The exchange of information between users, collaborative decision making, and the support of complex safety-critical processes will be critical to ensuring health IT operates as expected in health care settings. Unlike some of the other areas where such research is conducted (such as nuclear power plant operations and flying airplanes), medical applications have an additional complexity in that health professionals are treating multiple patients over the same time period and do not have the opportunity to land and finish one flight before having to think about the next one. Interfaces that support this "context switching" are essential, and not enough is known about them.

Also important to safe design and development of technologies is a better understanding of the tradeoffs between standardization and customization of health IT. While many users would like to modify health IT to fit their specific needs and health care environments, customization can make systems difficult to analyze. Customization can also prevent development of widespread solutions. On the other hand, health IT products that are too standardized may not appropriately fit into an organization's workflow. A similar argument is considered in our policy discussion about the tension between regulation and innovation. Rigorous scientific evidence ought to serve as the basis to achieve a balance between making things the same and letting them differ. Similarly, research is needed to address the mismatch between the assumptions of health IT designers and the actual clinical work environment.

IMPLEMENTATION AND USE OF TECHNOLOGIES

Evaluations of how safely health technologies are implemented and used will help build safer systems. There is a need to build a larger body of evidence that identifies the most successful implementation methods as well as to study and measure actual use of health IT. An area of particular concern also underrepresented in the literature is use of patient engagement tools.

To identify successful implementation methods, sharing of common experiences can help create guidance specific to the acquisition and initial implementation of health IT. For example, is the best method of implementing health IT to take a "big bang" approach where all divisions of an organization adopt a health IT product at the same time, or is it to roll out the product incrementally? Evidence for the best method to back up an EHR in case of unforeseen downtime and other types of contingency plans would help reduce the risks of making mistakes and thereby improve the overall system safety.

Further investigations will also be needed about how health IT products are actually being introduced and integrated into clinical workflows. Currently, data on the impact of health IT on workflows are sparse and largely anecdotal. Examining disruption of workflow can reveal where health IT design poorly matches the incentives and demands clinicians encounter during work, generating knowledge about the generic and specific nature of problems. Obstacles to sharing experiences gained during implementation include that providers are too busy to document what happened to them, and that experiences across both large and small medical service organizations are needed. Facilitating the lessons learned may require additional resources from a public source. Specific measures of usability that apply across clinicians and settings would help speed adoption. Assessments made after clinical implementation of health IT can evaluate whether or not it is working as designed as well as the presence of adverse events. Detailed measures will be needed to assess the actual performance of any life-critical technology. For example, measures on how well the technology has been implemented in the clinical setting could monitor whether a technology is being used safely and is not inadvertently introducing risks into the clinical workflow. Exploring the safety consequences of work-as-designed compared to work-as-practiced at the front lines of care delivery is crucial. For example, the Adverse Event Reporting System has been of great value in understanding the practical risks of drug administration.

Another critically important area for research is effective flow of information to both providers and patients. In an age where the average patient record weighs seven pounds, research is needed on summarization, saliency, and understanding to capture the nonlinear nature of the health care work environment (ACHE-NJ, 2009). Designing information presentation to minimize safety risks with minimum effort is still an unsolved problem. Information visualization is not as advanced in parts of clinical medicine as compared with other scientific disciplines.

Finally, use of health IT by patients needs to be evaluated. Patients are now engaging in their own care using an increasing number of diverse methods and tools, particularly with Internet-based applications. Learning how patients interact with these tools and their expectations for their care will be critical to achieve high levels of patient–clinician interaction as health care enters an era of ubiquitous computing. Understanding the impact of sharing electronic records and the effect of patient partnerships in owning and interacting with data, for example in a personal health record, can help improve safety. At the same time, patients often do not understand instructions given by medical or nursing staff, and do not follow them. To achieve greater safety, mechanisms will need to be developed between clinicians and patients to assess and verify patient- and caregiver-entered data to develop a shared understanding of how such data will be used. Interfaces that can help both patients and clinicians access and assess a patient's health data will become increasingly important. Any unintended effects of patient engagement tools also ought to be studied. Patient engagement tools might reduce health disparities and improve the health of populations. On the other hand, they might cause individuals to misinterpret their own results or to fret about insignificant changes in test results. Researchers will need to be cognizant of the array of patient engagement tools and monitor their effects on patient safety.

CONSIDERATIONS FOR RESEARCHERS

Some research questions about health IT and patient safety are suited for academic research. Manufacturers and health care organizations likely will not examine evaluation methods, considerations specific to small practices and hospitals, and the impact on population health.

Limitations in the quality of the literature arise in part from poor availability of high-quality data and adequately powered research methods. Study methods generally considered the gold standard in health care such as randomized controlled trials are often inappropriately applied to evaluations of health care because they are unable to consider the many exogenous factors facing complex systems. Research should exploit the methods of other disciplines such as those prevalent in social sciences. This is critical to studying the safety of health care systems and is particularly relevant to studying sociotechnical systems.

Further understanding of the various sociotechnical domains discussed in Chapter 3 will be essential, especially in the areas where domains overlap. Research on the influence of each domain on the quality and safety of care will be needed to identify system vulnerabilities and ways to address them. Any investigations about sociotechnical systems will require collaboration and learning from a wide collection of disciplines and industries, including systems engineering, human factors, IT, and health care, among others.

Studies of implementation need to be evaluated in situ to account for the many factors that affect health IT products as they are actually used. Research methods are currently limited and mostly test health IT products in vitro. Methods for in situ testing need to be developed, as in situ testing becomes increasingly valuable.

It will also be important to examine niche health IT products that are being developed for medical specialties such as anesthesia information systems, radiology information systems, and perioperative management systems. These systems and their interactions within EHRs are not yet widely reported in the literature but carry potentially great implications for patient safety.

Research today largely studies what happens in large hospitals. Additional study is needed of care delivered by small practices and hospitals and/ or providers in rural areas. Most U.S. medical care is provided by smaller providers. They have special problems related to staffing, workflow, and a safety culture not dependent on local IT expertise. Examples of research efforts specific to small providers include what type of staffing model best supports patient safety, characteristics of optimal workflow, and how to promote a culture of safety in these smaller organizations in the presence of health IT.

Population health is an area of great promise for health IT to improve patient safety and highlights the transformative potential of health IT. Preliminary experiences have found that the data generated by the use of health IT impacts population health. Specific to patient safety, EHR data might be used to identify close calls and adverse events at the community and population levels. Beyond patient safety, trends in health IT–generated data can create a pool for future research. For example, such data can lead to recognition that specific medications can have previously unknown risks or that widespread use of health IT can actually create larger disparities in care. While such studies were outside the committee's scope, inquiries at the population level ought to be considered as areas for further research.

To facilitate research, more data will be needed. All users and vendors of EHR technology could maintain records available (in anonymized form) for researchers. These records could be best used if sufficiently complete to support decision making for safety and to permit comparison of the risks and rewards of different strategies for design, implementation, and use. These data ought not to be used for either liability or disciplinary action.

POLICY ISSUES

The committee encountered a number of specific policy questions for which evidence was lacking, such as "Is health IT safe?" and "How safe is safe?". To inform better policy decisions, the effectiveness of regional extension centers, health information exchanges, and regional health information organizations needs to be measured.

The impact of oversight and regulation in the context of health IT and patient safety will require continual monitoring so that future policy decisions can have a base upon which to make informed decisions. This is especially important given the complexity of health IT. The intended and unintended consequences of policy decisions targeting health IT may have significant ramifications for the safety of care. For example, monetary incentives that encourage speed of installation above all else may cause inadequate and risky systems to be used. On the other hand, a monetary incentive for usability standards might produce safer patient care.

Another area for research is focusing on how to best achieve the maximum positive impact of health IT on safety. A better understanding of the unintended consequences will help us determine how to balance research investments by focusing on eliminating health IT–introduced errors or how to perfect and broadly disseminate features of health IT that lead to the greatest improvements in safety.

Understanding both the positive and negative unintended consequences will be critical to developing stronger, more effective policies. A summary of findings related to health IT policies ought to become part of an annual report submitted to the Secretary of Health and Human Services (HHS) on the safety of EHRs, EHR systems, and health IT capabilities in general.

The value proposition for health IT is beyond our scope, but it is poorly developed in the current literature. Costs for implementing and maintaining health IT can be extremely high and can be a deterrent to adopting technologies. On the other hand, health IT has been considered a tool to help potentially reduce health care costs in the long term. Clear evidence does not exist yet supporting one argument over another, and the lack of evidence is troubling for a technology that is so expensive and heavily privatized.

SUPPORTING FUTURE RESEARCH

While many of the above suggested research areas are not necessarily limited to health IT and can also apply to the paper-based world, the application of research to health IT is needed because of the widespread presence of health IT products in health care delivery. More research can foster more rapid improvements in patient safety (examples of future research ideas are shown in Box 7-1).

HHS should support a research program to study patient safety and the use of information technology with the goal of addressing the issues raised throughout this report. This research program should be carefully developed to ensure scientific rigor and thoughtful inquiry into the complex relationship between patient safety and the use of health IT. Within the department, a number of agencies such as the Agency for Healthcare Research and Quality (AHRQ), the Centers for Disease Control and Prevention, the Centers for Medicare & Medicaid Services, and the National Institutes of Health (through the National Library of Medicine) fund research on health IT and informatics. HHS could consider using demonstration projects to answer questions about the contribution of health IT to patient safety or using the Practice-based Research Networks to develop research and data about health IT implementation and use in primary care facilities. These should be part of a sustained, ongoing research program with substantial support for basic and applied research. It should be of a magnitude appropriate for such a large effort; comparable high-technology industries often spend 10 percent of their yearly revenue on research and development (NSF, 2011).

Many industries contribute to the research on improving technology safety and are supported by the government. In an effort to create a shared learning environment, a future research program should combine efforts from a cross-disciplinary set of organizations. For example, many state-based programs are driving innovation in health IT and should be leveraged. Additionally, agencies such as the Department of Defense, the Department of Energy, the Department of Veterans Affairs, the National Institute for Standards and Technology, and the National Science Foundation all support and/or conduct research in improving the safety of technology. These agencies are leaders in the area of technology safety research and their expertise should be leveraged for the development of safe health IT.

> Recommendation 10: HHS, in collaboration with other research groups, should support cross-disciplinary research toward the use of health IT as part of a learning health care system. Products of this research should be used to inform the design, testing, and use of health IT. Specific areas of research include
>
>   a. User-centered design and human factors applied to health IT;
>   b. Safe implementation and use of health IT by all users;
>   c. Sociotechnical systems associated with health IT; and
>   d. Impact of policy decisions on health IT use in clinical practice.

BOX 7-1
Examples of Productive Areas for Further Research

The work organization problem: Health IT typically focuses on individual patient details with little support for actual clinical work. How can IT be designed to better support the clinical work activities of health professionals? For example, can IT be used to track and schedule work tasks for clinicians and triage these as emergencies and delays accumulate through the day? Clinical work involves many levels of interruptions; how can health IT be designed to support clinicians in resuming interrupted work and in switching contexts to deal with an interruption? What sorts of status displays or other methods can help clinicians "see" the state of their work and recognize changing priorities and opportunities?

The information structure problem: Health IT designs usually do not reflect clinical associations when organizing and presenting data. Related medications, vital signs, and laboratory studies are routinely presented separately rather than in relation to each other. For example, hypertension appears separately from the current blood pressure and current or past medications, requiring the clinician to track data across various screens in order to synthesize an understanding of a patient's high blood pressure and its treatment. How can health IT be used to create meaningful representations of clinical data and knowledge?

The pick-list problem: Reports of wrong patient–wrong drug problems with health IT commonly arise from the pick-list problem. Health IT designs require practitioners to select single items from sometimes very long pick lists or menu lists, often containing similar terms presented in alphabetical order. There are lists of patients, lists of tests, lists of drugs, lists of results, and others. Health professionals struggle to find the desired entry in such lists and often select the wrong item, sometimes discovering this only much later. How can lists be presented so that their order and appearance make it easy to know what choices are available and easier to select the desired item?

The alarm/alert problem: Health professionals are drowning in data overload, and the current alarms and alerts within health IT often add to the problem. The "alarm problem" is generic and found across health IT and clinical practice. Each alert can be justified in isolation, but in combination these alerts can become a distraction. How can the use of alerts be managed at the system level so that clinicians receive useful alerts? For example, can the boundaries that trigger alerts be represented while orders are being entered so that clinicians do not have to "click through" multiple alerts after order entry? Can health IT track the presentation of alerts to specific clinicians so that alerts appear when medicines or conditions new to that clinician appear?

The cooperative work problem: Health IT typically treats activities as belonging to individual clinicians and as being accomplished serially, but clinicians often work in tandem or in small groups and communicate with each other about goals and task details. How can health IT be designed and configured to assist cooperative work?

The accountability and reimbursement problem: Health IT often incorporates features that serve accounting and reimbursement functions. Large parts of the clinical record are being generated to conform to billing requirements or to provide a stream of accountability information for later review. These functions are valuable but do not directly aid the clinical process and can make clinical care more difficult by demanding attention and hiding meaningful data with bureaucratic camouflage. What are the consequences for clinical care of including all these functions in health IT designs? Can health IT be configured to encourage recording of high-quality clinical observations rather than just the accumulation of clinically meaningless filler?

The availability problem: The benefits of health IT are often touted by vendors and chief information officers but outages are nearly always accompanied by statements that "no patient was harmed" by the computer breakdown. These characterizations are seemingly in conflict. What is the real impact of system outages? How often does this occur? How can the effects be determined?

The interoperability at the user level problem: Each health IT vendor has its own "look and feel" and individual implementations are customized so that each facility has unique features. Many health professionals work in more than one facility and encounter these different products on a regular basis. Is it possible to make health IT interoperable at the user level so that clinicians moving from one facility to another do not have to learn a new way of doing things each time? Can systems be designed so that clinician profiles developed in one system can be used in another? What are the consequences of having every implementation be different from every other implementation?

REFERENCES

ACHE-NJ (American College of Healthcare Executive of New Jersey). 2009. *EMRgency medicine: The impact of EMR/EHR on healthcare, Keynotes and expert panel discussion.* http://www.slideshare.net/sdorfman/emrgemcy-medicine-the-impact-of-emrehr-on-healthcare-keynotes-and-expert-panel-discussion-121009-in-nj (accessed July 9, 2011).
NSF (National Science Foundation). 2011. *Research and development in industry: 2006-2007.* http://www.nsf.gov/statistics/nsf11301/pdf/nsf11301.pdf (accessed July 25, 2011).

Appendix A

Glossary

Adverse event—An event resulting in unintended harm to a patient from a medical intervention (IOM, 2004)

Deployment—Phase when a health IT product is initially installed in a health care system

Implementation—Deployment and integration of a health IT product into clinical workflow

Interoperability—Ability for two or more systems or components to exchange information and to use the information that has been exchanged (IEEE, 1990)

Maintenance—Processes for manufacturers and health care organizations to sustain the good working condition of a health IT product and keep versions up to date

Metadata—Data describing attributes of the data themselves

Patient engagement tools—Technologies used primarily by patients to help them track, manage, and take part in their own health care

Performance requirements—A set of criteria delineating what a health IT product should achieve

Quality management principles and practices—A set of principles and practices an organization uses to improve performance and quality

Safe—Avoiding injuries to patients from the care that is intended to help them (IOM, 2001)

Sociotechnical systems—A construct identifying the interactions between people, processes, technology, organizations, and environment that influence complex systems

Usability—Extent to which a product can be used by specific users to achieve specified goals with effectiveness, efficiency, and satisfaction in a specific context of use (ISO, 1998)

Users—Health professionals, health care organizations, and patients who may actively use health IT products

Vendors—Companies that make, sell, and may provide support for health IT products and homegrown systems

REFERENCES

IEEE (Institute of Electrical and Electronics Engineers). 1990. *IEEE standard computer dictionary: A compilation of IEEE standard computer glossaries.* New York: IEEE.

IOM (Institute of Medicine). 2001. *Crossing the quality chasm: A new health system for the 21st century.* Washington, DC: National Academy Press.

IOM. 2004. *Patient safety: Achieving a new standard for care.* Washington, DC: The National Academies Press.

ISO (International Organization for Standardization). 1998. *International standard 9241 ergonomic requirements for office work with visual display terminals, part 11: Guidance on usability.* Geneva, Switzerland: ISO.

Appendix B

Literature Review Methods

The committee reviewed the published literature to identify what is known about the relationship between patient safety and health information technology (health IT)–assisted care. In the preliminary analysis, the literature was searched, reviewed, analyzed, sorted into categories (see category definitions below), and summarized into a table. "Health IT–assisted care" means health care and services that incorporate and take advantage of health IT and health information exchanges for the purpose of improving the processes and outcomes of health care services. Health IT–assisted care includes care supported by and involving electronic health records (EHRs), clinical decision support, computerized provider order entry, health information exchange, patient engagement technologies, and other health information technologies used in clinical care.

SEARCH STRATEGY

Extensive search terms were used in four databases—Medline, EMBase, Web of Science, and Cochrane—yielding initial results of 2,868 articles, books, and other literature. A search strategy was developed for each database using terms and Medical Subject Headings focused in subject areas related to patient safety, medical informatics, and other related areas.[1]

---

[1] Subject areas included quality of health care (accidental harm, adverse events, diagnostic errors, errors of omission or commission, injuries, medication errors, safety, and treatment outcomes) and medical informatics (human factors, informatics, system design, systems analysis, usability, and user–computer interface).

Strategy parameters included limiting the search to human subjects, the English language, and results published between January 2005 and November 2010 because the literature regarding health IT evolves rapidly and continually builds upon itself. Next, hand searches through the references were conducted and relevant studies were included. Primary and secondary research (e.g., meta-analyses, controlled trials) suggested by the public and the committee were also added to the search results. Other literature (e.g., editorials, commentaries) were excluded from the search results.

CATEGORIZATION AND ANALYSIS

Titles and abstracts of the articles produced from the search were rigorously reviewed to determine which studies met the inclusion criteria for study quality and relevance. Pairs of reviewers evaluated titles and abstracts of all studies within each subject area. Each reviewer independently assigned articles to one of three categories with Category 1 being the most relevant and Category 3 being the least relevant (see definitions below).

Category 1: Literature examining how health IT affects patient safety.

> 1a. Systematic reviews[2]
> 1b. Experimental studies
> 1c. Observational studies

Category 2: Literature describing efforts to improve quality of health care through implementation of one or more of the following components of health IT (e.g., system design, systems analysis, usability, user–computer interface, or human factors).

Category 3: Studies not related to patient safety and health IT.

Reviewers then compared their evaluations, and any disagreement was resolved through discussion. The full texts of articles determined to be Category 1 were retrieved, evaluated, and, if needed, recategorized.

---

[2] A systematic review is defined as a scientific investigation that focuses on a specific question and that uses explicit, preplanned scientific methods to identify, select, assess, and summarize the findings of similar but separate studies. It may or may not include a quantitative synthesis of the results from separate studies (meta-analysis).

RESULTS

The search yielded 128 Category 1 articles. These articles were then placed in two tables—one table summarizing each of the systematic reviews (Table B-1)[3] and the other table summarizing each of the experimental and observational studies (Table B-2).[4] Within the table, the articles were then organized by the type of health IT component.[5]

An additional 479 articles were identified as Category 2, which inform broader parameters of patient safety and health IT. These parameters include efforts to improve quality of health care through the implementation of one or more of the following: system design, systems analysis, usability, user–computer interface, or human factors.

The remaining studies were classified as Category 3 studies, which did not meet the inclusion criteria and were not broadly considered in the literature review or table.

Although Category 1 articles published before January 2005 and Category 2 articles were not included in the literature review table, these articles were used throughout the committee's deliberations as background. Additionally, articles that were not studies or reviews of studies, such as editorials and commentaries, were not included in the literature table but were still considered and used in the analysis of the report.

---

[3] Table B-1 is included on CD in the back of the book and online at: http://www.nap.edu/html/13269/app_b_tables.pdf.

[4] Table B-2 is included on CD in the back of the book and online at: http://www.nap.edu/html/13269/app_b_tables.pdf.

[5] The majority of the studies focused on how individual components of health IT affect patient safety (e.g., alerts, bar-coding, clinical decision support, EHRs, electronic prescribing, patient engagement tools, smartpumps, surveillance tools, and other health IT–assisted care). Therefore, the tables were organized by the components that each article was studying. Articles not focusing on a specific component were placed at the beginning of each table and are labeled as "overview" articles.

Appendix C

Abstract of "Roadmap for Provision of Safer Healthcare Information Systems: Preventing e-Iatrogenesis"[1]

Joan S. Ash, Ph.D., M.L.S., M.B.A.; Charles M. Kilo, M.D., M.P.H.;
Michael Shapiro, M.A., M.S.; Joseph Wasserman, B.A.;
Carmit McMullen, Ph.D.; William Hersh, M.D.

BACKGROUND AND METHODS

e-Iatrogenesis, defined as "patient harm caused at least in part by the application of health information technology" (Weiner et al., 2007), is of increasing concern as more and more hospitals are implementing health information systems (HIS). This report assesses how HIS can be designed, developed, implemented, monitored, and maintained to maximize safety. We specifically focus on hospital electronic health records (EHRs), clinical decision support (CDS), and computerized provider order entry (CPOE) systems. This white paper is intended to provide background for an Institute of Medicine (IOM) report on how the use of health information technology affects the safety of patient care by answering the following IOM-posed questions:

- What are the risks of health care information systems that arise from workflow and related issues?
- How have organizations acted to implement health care information systems safely?
- What are the impacts of customization on safety?
- What is the industry approach to managing change and customization?

A recent literature review by Harrington et al. (2011) has summarized the EHR safety literature, so we first reviewed all papers cited in their

---

[1] Full commissioned paper is included on the CD in the back of the book.

report. Of their 43 references, we identified 37 that were relevant to the scope of this article. We analyzed the bibliographies of these selected papers and performed a reverse bibliography search on the articles deemed most relevant and published since 2000. In total, we identified more than 100 sources relevant to the scope of this report. We then targeted topics for which published evidence was lacking and conducted several interviews with experts to help fill the knowledge gaps.

RESULTS

What Are the Risks of Health Information Systems That Arise from Workflow and Related Issues?

We found seven publications (Chuo and Hicks, 2008; Joint Commission on Accreditation of Healthcare Organizations, 2008; Magrabi et al., 2010; Myers et al., 2011; Santell et al., 2009; Walsh et al., 2006; Zhan et al., 2006) presenting results of assessments of e-iatrogenic risk. All are studies of large databases of reported errors, and they consistently indicate low levels of HIS-related risk, less than 1 percent of all errors. All point to the need for human diligence when using HIS. Specifically, they indicate that HIS-related errors are due to inadequate staffing levels, lack of user experience, mislabeled bar-codes on medications, human distraction, inaccurate data entry, system downtime, and missing data.

How Have Organizations Acted to Implement Health Information Systems Safely?

Prior to implementation, health care organizations can mitigate risk. There is a large literature base devoted to the risks inherent in commercial EHR systems, and also warnings about their impact on workflow. Many publications offer guidance to hospitals about assessing workflow, selecting systems for purchase, conducting simulation tests, training, and other mechanisms for ensuring safe HIS implementation. Numerous publications exist to guide the implementation process itself, but there are also several pointing to the risks of rapid implementation without appropriate preparation. Finally, after implementation, continuous monitoring and improvement can mitigate safety risks.

What Are the Impacts of Customization on Safety?

The literature indicates that customization of the EHR to fit local situations seems to be necessary for many reasons, but there is scant research on how much customization or what form of customization is needed to optimize EHR use and what the risks are from either too much or too little customization. The content of CDS likewise needs adaptation, especially to avoid alert fatigue. Any customization must be done with care so that system upgrades can be accommodated.

What Is the Industry Approach to Managing Change and Customization?

The current industry approach is fragmented; a report sponsored by the Agency for Healthcare Research and Quality describes a wide variety of vendor practices related to usability of systems (McDonnell et al., 2010). Because purchasers must usually customize systems to fit local workflows and regulations, HIS safety depends on a combination of industry and local diligence.

RECOMMENDATIONS

Although current evidence is limited, the presence of HIS appears to contribute to less than 1 percent of total errors in health care settings. However, indirect effects from disruption of workflow are difficult to measure. Further investigation into these issues is needed as soon as possible so that solid evidence can inform the bolus of HIS implementations in hospitals resulting from meaningful use regulations. In addition, expert consensus-based recommendations would be highly useful.

REFERENCES

Chuo, J., and R. W. Hicks. 2008. Computer-related medication errors in neonatal intensive care units. *Clinics in Perinatology* 35:119-139.

Joint Commission on Accreditation of Healthcare Organizations. 2008. Safely implementing health information and converging technologies. *Sentinel Event Alert* 42:1-4.

Harrington, L., D. Kennerly, and C. Johnson. 2011. Safety issues related to the electronic medical record (EMR): Synthesis of the literature from the last decade, 2000–2009. *Journal of Healthcare Management* 56(1):31-44.

Magrabi, F., M.-S. Ong, W. Runciman, and E. Coiera. 2010. An analysis of computer-related patient safety incidents to inform the development of a classification. *Journal of the American Medical Informatics Association* 17:663-670.

McDonnell, C., K. Werner, and L. Wendel. May, 2010. Electronic health record usability: Vendor practices and perspectives. AHRQ Publication No. 09(10)-0091-3-EF. Rockville, MD: Agency for Healthcare Research and Quality.

Myers, R. B., S. L. Jones, and D. F. Sittig. 2011. Review of reported clinical information system adverse events in U.S. Food and Drug Administration databases. *Applied Clinical Informatics* 2:63-74.

Santell, J. P., J. G. Kowiatek, R. J. Weber, R. W. Hicks, and C. A. Sirio. 2009. Medication errors resulting from computer entry by nonprescribers. *American Journal of Health-System Pharmacists* 66:843-853.

Walsh, K. E., W. G. Adams, H. Bauchner, R. J. Vinci, J. B. Chessare, M. R. Cooper, P. M. Hebert, E. G. Schainker, and C. P. Landrigan. 2006. Medication errors related to computerized order entry for children. *Pediatrics* 118(5):1872-1879.

Weiner, J. P., T. Kfuri, K. Chan, and J. B. Fowles. 2007. "E-iatrogenesis": The most critical unintended consequence of CPOE and other HIT. *Journal of the American Medical Informatics Association* 14(3):387-388.

Zhan, C., R. W. Hicks, C. M. Blanchette, M. A. Keyes, and D. D. Cousins. 2006. Potential benefits and problems with computerized prescriber order entry: Analysis of a voluntary medication error-reporting database. *American Journal of Health-System Pharmacists* 63:353-358.

Appendix D

Abstract of "The Impact of Regulation on Innovation in the United States: A Cross-Industry Literature Review"[1]

Luke A. Stewart

INTRODUCTION

Through a high-level, multi-industry review of the literature, this paper describes how regulation can both stifle and encourage innovation. The impact of regulation on innovation depends largely on the breadth and type of the regulation.

REGULATION AND INNOVATION

Innovation—the commercially successful application of an idea from invention, the initial development of a new idea, and the widespread adoption of the innovation—is classified by whether the innovation benefits the market or social welfare. *Market innovation* typically benefits producers, consumers, and society at large, although there are cases where it may only benefit producers at the expense of social welfare. *Social innovation* refers to product and process innovations that create social benefits, such as cleaner air, which firms cannot directly capture through market sales.

Firms can also choose to innovate incrementally or radically. *Incremental innovation* occurs when firms make relatively minor improvements to existing products and processes to comply with regulation. *Radical innovation* occurs when a firm replaces existing products or processes to comply with regulation. This type of innovation is costly and risky; however, it can yield greater benefits than incremental innovation.

---

[1] Full commissioned paper is included on the CD in the back of the book.

189

Like innovation, regulations can be economic or social in nature. *Economic regulation* sets market conditions; it often changes the market efficiency and potentially affects the equality and fairness of the market. *Social regulation*, on the other hand, seeks to protect the welfare of society or the environment. When the scope of regulation is narrow, firms may choose to change their products or processes so that they are no longer within the scope of the regulation, also known as *circumventive innovation*. When the scope of the regulation is broad, firms may prefer to change its product or process to adhere to the regulation—otherwise known as *compliance innovation*.

A regulation's stringency, flexibility, and effect on available market information—collectively known as *innovation dimensions* of regulation—can have drastic impacts on innovation. *Stringency* is the degree to which a regulation requires compliance innovation and imposes a compliance burden on a firm, industry, or market. Generally, the more stringent a regulation is, the more radical compliance innovation is required. Thus, stringent regulation increases risk, cost, and the chances of "dud" products or processes. *Flexibility* describes the number of implementation paths firms have available for compliance. *Information* measures whether a regulation promotes more or less complete information in the market. Although flexibility and increased available information generally aid innovation (see Table D-1), regulation or the possibility of regulation can induce two types of uncertainty—policy and compliance uncertainty.

Policy uncertainty occurs when a firm anticipates the enactment of a regulation at some time in the future and may cause firms to divert resources in preparation for future compliance. The degree of resources diverted depends on the anticipated stringency of the future regulation. Policy uncertainty may cause firms to innovate, even if regulations never become enacted. *Compliance uncertainty* is uncertainty caused by an existing regulation. This generally occurs when a firm does not know whether a product or process will comply with preexisting regulation or how much time is needed for the product or process to comply.

FINDINGS AND CONCLUSIONS

While it was found that the degree by which regulation affects innovation is highly variable and case specific, several common themes emerged:

- Policy uncertainty affects expected future regulation and can stifle innovation.
- Flexible regulations generally aid both market and social innovation.
- More complete market information aids innovation.
- Economic regulation tends to stifle market innovation.

TABLE D-1
Selected Attributes of Regulations and Their Theoretical Impacts on Innovation

Regulation	Compliance Burden	Compliance Innovation	
		"Dud" Inventions	Innovation
Flexibility			
Command and control	Higher	–	–
Incentives based	Lower	–	–
Specification standards	Higher	More	–
Performance standards	Lower	Less	–
Information			
Compliance value added	Lower	Lower	–
Compliance uncertainty	Higher	–	–
Stringency			
Moving target	Lower	Less	None/ Incremental
Disruptive regulation	Higher	More	Radical

- Social regulation tends to stimulate social innovation; however, more often than not, it stifles market innovation.
- Some evidence suggests more stringent and disruptive social regulation promotes more radical innovation, while the "moving target approach" of gradually increasing stringency over time results in incremental innovation.
- Regulation that does not require innovation for compliance will generally stifle innovation, although it may spur circumventive innovation if the firm or industry can find a path to escape the regulatory constraints.
- Regulation that does require compliance innovation has an unclear impact on innovation.
- A tradeoff exists between market innovation that benefits the firms and that which serves only to meet the compliance standards of regulation.

Appendix E

Dissenting Statement:
Health IT Is a Class III Medical Device

Richard I. Cook, M.D.

This appendix is a dissenting statement from committee member Richard Cook, and contains his alternate recommendation for the regulation of health IT.

Recommendation 9: The Secretary of Health and Human Services (HHS) should direct the Food and Drug Administration (FDA) to exercise its authority to regulate health IT, including all electronic health records (EHRs) and associated components, and health information exchanges, as Class III medical devices.

Medical and diagnostic devices have produced a therapeutic revolution, but in doing so they have also become more complex and less easily understood by those who use them. When well designed, well made, and properly used they support and lengthen life. If poorly designed, poorly made, and improperly used they can threaten and impair it. (President Gerald Ford, signing statement for Medical Device Amendments, May 28, 1976)

RATIONALE

Proponents and critics agree that health IT plays an important role in patient care and patient safety. Rather than being an adjunct or appendage of health care delivery, health IT is necessarily intimately woven into the fabric of patient care. Electronic medical records, digital imaging, provider order entry, and test results delivery do not "have an effect" on core medical functions; they *are* core medical functions. In contrast with, for example, electronic medical textbooks, health IT involves the generation, manipulation, storage, and display of patient- and provider-*specific* data. This need for specificity imposes special requirements on information technology. When a provider reads a laboratory result from the computer screen or enters an order for a medicine by mouse or keyboard, the patient context matters a great deal.

Until now, health IT's quality, accuracy, precision, reliability, and safety have been left almost entirely to vendors. Although facilities and, to a lesser extent, users can configure and adapt health IT for their own uses, as a practical matter it is the vendors who control what health IT looks like and how it performs. While this may be reasonable for consumer or even some commercial software and hardware, it is unacceptable for health IT that must provide high-level performance in a hazardous environment. Medical practice is inherently hazardous and devices used to care for patients are regulated.

Is health IT a medical device? If so, in the United States, FDA is charged with its regulation. According to law, a medical device is

> . . . an instrument, apparatus, implement, machine, contrivance, implant, in vitro reagent, or other similar or related article, including any component, part, or accessory, which is—
>
> (1) recognized in the official National Formulary, or the United States Pharmacopeia, or any supplement to them,
>
> (2) intended for use in the diagnosis of disease or other conditions, or in the cure, mitigation, treatment, or prevention of disease, in man or other animals, or
>
> (3) intended to affect the structure or any function of the body of man or other animals, and which does not achieve its primary intended purposes through chemical action within or on the body of man or other animals and which is not dependent upon being metabolized for the achievement of its primary intended purposes. (Federal Food, Drug, and Cosmetic Act, 21 U.S.C. § 321 SEC. 201)

Health IT components include items such as computerized provider order entry (CPOE), electronic medical records (EMRs), or EHRs. These components participate directly in diagnosis, cure, mitigation, treatment, and prevention of specified individual human beings. Health IT is a medical device and FDA is or should be its regulatory body.

The 1976 Medical Device Amendments to the Federal Food, Drug, and Cosmetic Act established three regulatory classes for medical devices. Class I devices are the simplest and are least likely to cause direct or indirect harm. The *tongue depressor* is a Class I device (its entry is in the Code of Federal Regulations at 21 CFR 880.6230). Class II devices include devices more likely to present some risk of harm. The *hearing aid* is a Class II device (21 CFR 801.420). The amendments define a Class III device as "one that supports or sustains human life or is of substantial importance in preventing impairment of human health or presents a potential, unreasonable risk of illness or injury." Class III includes obvious high-risk devices such as external cardiac defibrillators (21 CFR 870.5310) but also includes HIV tests (21 CFR 864.4020).

What class of medical device is health IT? Because some health IT device characteristics may require a different approach to regulation than is practical under current classification rules, perhaps health IT should have its own classification. Under existing rules, however, I believe that health IT should be classified as a Class III medical device for at least three reasons.

First, health IT functionality is widely regarded as essential for safe care. The proponents and vendors of health IT regularly and consistently point to the safety afforded by the use of health IT. According to the Institute of Medicine (IOM), human clinician errors are a major cause of morbidity and mortality (IOM, 1999). Preventing human clinician errors is one of the main functions of health IT and a primary rationale for the $32 billion investment in health IT committed by the Recovery Act of 2009. This surely makes health IT of "substantial importance in preventing impairment of human health," which is the central criterion of a Class III device.

Second, adoption of health IT has pervasive effects on basic health care delivery. Its use affects virtually every activity that takes place in a hospital, clinic, or doctor's office. Health IT receives, stores, and displays clinical information. It accepts, validates, and transmits orders for care and treatment. It notifies physicians, nurses, pharmacists, and technicians of patient conditions. It tracks clinical actions and assessments. These are not trivial functions, and their accuracy and reliability have direct impact on virtually every patient's well-being. Adopting health IT amounts to putting all the clinical eggs in a single basket. Unlike other medical devices, most of which have effects on a few hundred or thousand patients, health IT is on track to be *a medical device used for every person in the United States.*

The third reason it is a Class III device is that health IT can *and does* cause significant harm to patients. At least a few U.S. citizens—perhaps more than a few—have died or been maimed because of health IT. The extent of the injuries generated by health IT is unknown because no one has bothered to look for them in a systematic fashion. Indeed the failure to treat health IT as a medical device has played a significant role in keeping the problems with health IT from becoming known. Medical device manufacturers are obligated to report instances of patient harm connected to their devices. Health IT vendors are not. Problems and the resulting hazards from health IT cannot be addressed and fixed without first being identified through some form of reporting. The government's failure to treat health IT as a medical device has allowed manufacturers to keep the problems with health IT hidden and has made it possible for vendors to require contractual "gag clauses" that restrict open discussion of its problems.

Simply declaring health IT to be a medical device—even a Class III medical device—will not rectify the safety problem that health IT creates. It will, however, begin to bring this burgeoning area out of the shadows and into the light. This is a necessary part of improving its impact on patient safety.

Accidents involving health IT are complex events that require substantial forensic skill to detect and describe. The impact of health IT on system safety is most easily understood in cases of overt computer outages (sometimes described as system "crashes"), which deny clinicians access to the data and communications that these systems usually provide. Absurdly, when such an outage becomes public knowledge the system owners uniformly declare that "no patient was harmed." If so, the case for health IT must be weak indeed. There are presently no standards for assessing or reporting such outages or for judging their effects on safety.

But most of the impact of health IT on safety must be more subtle than the overt computer crash. The "copy forward" case described in Box E-1 is more representative. Here, data appear out of context and are misinterpreted. The simple existence of a datum inside a database does not ensure that its significance will be appreciated. Similarly, the appreciation of a datum in one circumstance does not ensure that it will be appreciated in all circumstances. Problems with "pick lists"—e.g., menus of medications, procedures, or laboratory tests—are common in other areas and also appear in reports of difficulties with health IT. It is remarkably easy to select the wrong patient or the wrong drug from these lists.

We know this not so much from studies of health IT as from experience in other domains. Indeed this experience is the basis for modern methods

---

BOX E-1

An abdominal ultrasound report in an electronic record appeared to indicate a blighted ovum, and a dilation and curettage (D&C) was performed a few days later. The patient returned to the ER [emergency room] 4 weeks after the D&C with abdominal pain. Repeat ultrasound revealed a 21-week pregnancy. A damaged fetus was delivered at 26 weeks. The ultrasound result had actually been obtained several weeks prior to the date of the record in which it appeared. The report had been copied forward into that record and appeared out of context.

for IT designs for use in hazardous settings. It is not surprising that such events are now being discovered in health IT. *What is surprising is that those creating and promoting these large systems have neither anticipated them nor looked for them.* The development of health IT is marked by an optimism about the effects of IT that are unwarranted and naive. And the willingness to embrace this optimism to the extent of making large-scale investments in these systems and only later asking what their impact might be on patient safety borders on recklessness.

Mounting an effort to bring device regulation to health IT will be challenging and demands both added resources and new methodologies for FDA. It is clear from a recent IOM report (IOM, 2011) that medical device regulation itself will benefit from careful review and revision. But make no mistake: health IT is a medical device. It should be regulated as a medical device now and should have been regulated as a medical device in the past.

REFERENCES

IOM (Institute of Medicine). 1999. *To err is human: Building a safer health system.* Washington, DC: National Academy Press.

IOM. 2011. *Medical devices and the public's health: The FDA 510(k) clearance process at 35 years.* Washington, DC: The National Academies Press.

Appendix F

Committee Member and
Staff Biographies

COMMITTEE BIOGRAPHIES

Gail L. Warden, M.H.A., FACHE (*Chair*), president emeritus of Detroit-based Henry Ford Health System, served as its president and chief executive officer from April 1988 to 2003. Prior to this role, Mr. Warden served as president and chief executive officer of Group Health Cooperative of Puget Sound as well as executive vice president of the American Hospital Association. He serves as a director of Picker Institute Inc. He has been a director of National Research Corp. since January 2005. He served as a director of Comerica Inc. from July 2000 to December 31, 2006. Mr. Warden serves in numerous leadership positions, as chairman to several national health care committees and as board member to many other health care–related committees and institutions. In addition, he is a professor of health management and policy for the University of Michigan School of Public Health. He serves the Detroit, Michigan, community through various memberships on local governing committees and groups. Mr. Warden received an honorary doctorate in public administration from Central Michigan University and an honorary doctorate of humane letters from Rosalind Franklin University of Medicine and Science, a master of hospital administration from the University of Michigan, and a bachelor of arts from Dartmouth College.

James P. Bagian, M.D., is the director of the Center for Healthcare Engineering and Patient Safety and is a professor in the Medical School and the College of Engineering at the University of Michigan. Previously, he served as the first director of the Department of Veterans Affairs (VA) National

Center for Patient Safety (NCPS) and the first chief Patient Safety Officer for the VA from 1999 to 2010, where he developed numerous patient safety–related tools and programs that have been adopted nationally and internationally. Dr. Bagian served as a NASA astronaut and is a veteran of two Space Shuttle missions including as the lead mission specialist for the first dedicated Life Sciences Spacelab mission. His primary interest and expertise involves the development and implementation of multidisciplinary programs and projects that involve the integration of engineering, medical and life sciences, and human factor disciplines. Presently, he is applying the majority of his attention to the application of systems engineering approaches to the analysis of medical adverse events and the development and implementation of suitable corrective actions that will enhance patient safety primarily through preventive means. He received his B.S. in mechanical engineering from Drexel University and his M.D. from Jefferson Medical College at Thomas Jefferson University. Dr. Bagian was elected to both the National Academy of Engineering and the Institute of Medicine (IOM) and has served on or chaired numerous National Research Council (NRC) and IOM committees.

David W. Bates, M.D., M.Sc., is the director of the Center for Patient Safety Research and Practice at Brigham and Women's Hospital, where he is the chief of the Division of General Medicine. He is also the medical director of clinical and quality analysis, information systems (IS). He is a professor in medicine at Harvard Medical School and has a joint appointment at the Harvard School of Public Health in the Department of Health Policy and Management. He serves as one of the directors of the clinical effectiveness program. He is also external program lead for research for the World Alliance for Patient Safety of the World Health Organization. Dr. Bates received his B.S. degree in chemistry from Stanford University, his M.D. from Johns Hopkins School of Medicine, and his M.Sc. in health policy and management from the Harvard School of Public Health. Dr. Bates's primary informatics interest has been the use of computer systems to improve patient care, especially with respect to clinical decision support. He has done extensive work on evaluating the incidence and prevention of adverse drug events. Another area of focus has been on improving efficiency and quality using information systems with regards to diagnostic testing. He also has done a series of studies focusing on health information technology policy.

Dedra Cantrell, R.N., B.S.N., M.S., C.P., is the chief information officer of Emory Healthcare, Inc., in Atlanta, Georgia. Emory Healthcare is an integrated academic health care system committed to caring for patients and their families, educating health care professionals for the future, pursuing discovery research and clinical innovation, and serving its community. The clinical arm of the Woodruff Health Sciences Center of Emory University, Emory Healthcare is the largest, most comprehensive health system in the state of Georgia. Ms. Cantrell earned her bachelor's degree in nursing from Brenau University and worked as a registered nurse in multiple capacities before becoming involved in health care information technology. She went to Emory in 1994 as director of Patient Services Information Systems for the Emory University Hospital and then moved the following year to become a senior business analyst in the Emory Healthcare Information Services Department. Ms. Cantrell was promoted to director of client and application services in 1996, named executive director of Emory Healthcare Information Services in 1998, and was promoted to chief information officer in 2000. Ms. Cantrell recently earned her master's degree in organizational management from Capella University.

David C. Classen, M.D., M.S., is an associate professor of medicine at the University of Utah and an active consultant in infectious diseases at the University of Utah School of Medicine in Salt Lake City, and he is also a senior partner at CSC. He served as chief medical resident at the University of Connecticut. He is board certified in internal medicine and infectious diseases. He was the chair of Intermountain Healthcare's clinical quality committee for drug use and evaluation and was the initial developer of patient safety research and patient safety programs at Intermountain Healthcare. In addition he developed, implemented, and evaluated a computerized physician order entry program at LDS Hospital that significantly improved the safety of medication use. He was a member of the IOM committee that developed the National Healthcare Quality Report and was also a member of the IOM committee on patient safety data standards. He chaired the QUIC (federal safety taskforce)/Institute for Healthcare Improvement (IHI) collaborative on improving safety in high-hazard areas. Dr. Classen was co-chair of the IHI's collaborative on perioperative safety and the surgical safety collaborative. He was also a faculty member of the IHI/National Health Foundation Safer Patients Initiative in the United Kingdom. In addition, Dr. Classen is a developer of the "Trigger Tool Methodology" at IHI, used for the improved detection of adverse events, which is currently being used by more than 500 different health care organizations throughout the United States and Europe. Dr. Classen also leads the development and publication of the new compendium of strategies for the prevention of health care–associated infections jointly released by the Infectious Disease Society of America, the Society of Healthcare Epidemiology, The Joint Commission, the American Hospital Association, and the Association of Practitioners of Infection Control. He currently co-chairs the National Quality Forum's (NQF's) patient safety common formats committee and is an advisor to the Leapfrog Group and has developed and implemented the computerized provider order entry (CPOE)/EHR flight simulator for the Leapfrog Group and the NQF. This EHR flight simulator has been used to evaluate hundreds of inpatient and ambulatory EHR systems after implementation across the United States and the United Kingdom. He received his M.D. from the University of Virginia School of Medicine and an M.S. in medical informatics from the University of Utah School of Medicine.

Richard I. Cook, M.D., is a physician, educator, and researcher at the University of Chicago. His current research interests include the study of human error, the role of technology in human expert performance, and patient safety. He worked in the computer industry in supercomputer system design and engineering applications and later received his M.D. from the University of Cincinnati. Since November 1994, he has been faculty in the Department of Anesthesia and Intensive Care of the University of Chicago. Dr. Cook has investigated a variety of safety issues in such diverse areas as urban mass transportation, semiconductor manufacturing, and military software systems. He is often a consultant for not-for-profit organizations, government agencies, and academic groups. His noteworthy publications include "Gaps in the Continuity of Patient Care and Progress in Patient Safety," "Operating at the Sharp End: The Complexity of Human Error," "Adapting to New Technology in the Operating Room," and the monograph *A Tale of Two Stories: Contrasting Views of Patient Safety.*

Don E. Detmer, M.D., M.A., is medical director of advocacy and health policy of the American College of Surgeons, professor emeritus and professor of medical education in the Department of Public Health Sciences at the University of Virginia, and visiting professor at the College of Healthcare Information Management Executives (CHIME), University College of London. Dr. Detmer is a member of the IOM as well as a lifetime associate of the National Academies, a fellow of the American Association for the Advancement of Science as well as the American Colleges of Medical Informatics, Sports Medicine, and Surgeons. Dr. Detmer is immediate past president of American Medical Informatics Association (AMIA), past chairman of the Board on Health Care Services and the membership committee of the IOM, the National Committee on Vital and Health Statistics, and the board of regents of the National Library of Medicine (NLM). He was a member of the national Commission on Systemic Interoperability. He chaired the 1991 IOM study *The Computer-Based Patient Record* and co-edited the 1997 version of the same report. He was a member of the committee that developed the IOM reports *To Err Is Human* and *Crossing the Quality Chasm.* His education includes an M.D. from the University of Kansas and an M.A. from the University of Cambridge. Dr. Detmer's research interests include national health information policy, quality improvement, compartment syndromes, and management of academic health centers. He has written and edited a number of research articles, books, book chapters, and monographs on these topics.

Meghan Dierks, M.D., is assistant professor of medicine, Harvard Medical School, in the Division of Clinical Informatics at Beth Israel Deaconess Medical Center in Boston, Massachusetts. She also holds a position of director of clinical systems analysis at Beth Israel Deaconess Medical Center. In these roles, Dr. Dierks conducts a broad range of both operational and research activities in the areas of clinical systems analysis, risk analysis, decision analysis, and human factors engineering (emphasis on cognitive engineering and macroergonomics). Dr. Dierks is a board-certified general surgeon who trained at Washington University, St. Louis, Missouri, and the Lahey Clinic, Burlington, Massachusetts. She completed the Harvard-Massachusetts Institute of Technology (MIT) program in biomedical informatics supported by an NLM training grant and was the Douglas Porter Fellow in Informatics at the Beth Israel Deaconess Medical Center. She has a baccalaureate degree from Brown University and an M.D. from the University of Texas Health Science Center–Houston. In addition to her academic position at Harvard Medical School, she has been a visiting scholar and research affiliate at MIT and is an adjunct faculty at the University of Maryland Division of Reliability Engineering. She is a former executive medical director for GE Healthcare IT, where she provided clinical input to design controls and was responsible for risk analysis. In her role as executive medical director, Dr. Dierks also held a leadership role in clinical research operations across all of GE Healthcare. Dr. Dierks spent 3 years with the Food and Drug Administration's (FDA's) Center for Devices and Radiological Health working on a range of cross-departmental projects under the deputy director that focused on risk analysis, mitigation, and strategic planning around medical devices shortages.

Terhilda Garrido, M.P.H., is vice president, health information technology transformation and analytics, within the national quality and care delivery organization at Kaiser Permanente. Her team is responsible for realizing the strategic value and maximizing opportunities for Kaiser Permanente's electronic health record. She also currently co-leads Kaiser Permanente's efforts to qualify for "meaningful use." Her areas of focus include evaluation of new EHR–based innovations, strategic impact of personal health records (PHRs)/EHRs, the business case for Kaiser Permanente's investment, leveraging health IT to improve quality, patient safety, efficiency, and equity. She has published on these topics and lends her expertise to various organizations within the health care industry. Prior to joining Kaiser, she did economic modeling and consulting for the European Economic Community and others. Ms. Garrido holds an operations research degree in engineering from Princeton University and a master's degree in public health in biostatistics from University of California at Berkeley. She completed graduate work at the Colegio de Mexico, Mexico City.

Ashish Jha, M.D., M.P.H., is an associate professor of health policy and management at the Harvard School of Public Health and an associate professor of medicine at Harvard Medical School. He is also an associate physician at Boston's Brigham and Women's Hospital and VA Boston Healthcare System. Over the past 3 years, he has served as special advisor for quality and safety to the VA. Dr. Jha received his M.D. from Harvard Medical School in 1997 and trained in internal medicine at the University of California, San Francisco, where he also served as chief medical resident. He completed his general medicine fellowship from Brigham and Women's Hospital and Harvard Medical School and received his M.P.H. in clinical effectiveness from the Harvard School of Public Health in 2004. He joined the faculty in July 2004. Dr. Jha is a practicing general internist with a clinical focus on hospital care. The major themes of his research include (1) quality of care provided by health care systems with a focus on safety, efficiency, and effectiveness; (2) health information technology as a tool to reduce disparities and improve the quality, efficiency, and safety of care; (3) disparities in care, with a focus on the quality of care provided by minority-serving providers; and (4) hospital governance and its impact on quality of care.

Michael Lesk, Ph.D., is professor of library and information science at Rutgers University and past department chair (2005-2008). After receiving a Ph.D. in chemical physics, Dr. Lesk joined the computer science research group at Bell Laboratories, and from 1984 to 1995 managed computer science research at Bellcore. He was then head of the division of information and intelligent systems at the National Science Foundation (1998-2002), and then joined Rutgers. He is best known for work in electronic libraries, and his book *Practical Digital Libraries* was published in 1997 by Morgan Kaufmann and the revision *Understanding Digital Libraries* appeared in 2004. His research has included the CORE project for chemical information, and he wrote some Unix system utilities including those for table printing (tbl), lexical analyzers (lex), and intersystem mail (uucp). His other technical interests include document production and retrieval software, computer networks, computer languages, and human–computer interfaces. He is a fellow of the Association for Computing Machinery, received the Flame award from the Usenix association, and in 2005 was elected to the National Academy of Engineering. He chairs the NRC board on research data and information.

Arthur Aaron Levin, M.P.H., is co-founder and the director of the Center for Medical Consumers, a New York City–based nonprofit organization committed to informed consumer and patient health care decision making, patient safety, evidence-based, high-quality medicine, and health care system transparency. Mr. Levin was a member of the IOM committee on the quality of health care that published the *To Err Is Human* and *Crossing the Quality Chasm* reports. Mr. Levin also was a member of the committee that issued an IOM letter report in October 2007, *Opportunities for Coordination and Clarity to Advance the National Health Information Agenda*, and served on the committee that wrote *Knowing What Works in Health Care: A Roadmap for the Nation* published in fall 2008. He is a former member of the IOM's Board for Health Care Services. He is currently serving as chair of the NQF Consensus Standards Approval Committee and is co-chair of the National Committee for Quality Assurance (NCQA) Committee on Performance Measures. Mr. Levin ended 4 years of service on FDA's Drug Safety and Risk Management Advisory Committee (DSaRM) in May 2007 and continues to serve on select FDA advisory committees as a consultant expert in drug safety and risk management representing consumers. He also serves on the boards of the Foundation for Informed Medical Decision Making and the Citizens Advocacy Center in Washington. Mr. Levin is a member of the board of directors and the executive committee of the New York eHealth Collaborative (NYeC) a not-for-profit, multistakeholder organization. NYeC was created to provide and support a governance process that provides policy direction to New York State's HEAL investment of more than $200 million dedicated to advancing health IT and health information exchange (HIE). NYeC is also the recipient (on behalf of the state) of more than $50 million in HIE and regional extension center (REC) grants from the Office of the National Coordinator. Mr. Levin earned his M.P.H. in health policy from Columbia University School of Public Health and a B.A. in philosophy from Reed College.

John R. Lumpkin, M.D., M.P.H., is the senior vice president and the director of the Robert Wood Johnson Foundation's health care group, where he is responsible for the overall planning, budgeting, staffing, management, and evaluation of all program and administrative activities. Before joining the Foundation in April 2003, Lumpkin served as director of the Illinois Department of Public Health for 12 years. During his more than 17 years with the department, he served as acting director and prior to that as associate director. Dr. Lumpkin is a member of the IOM of the National Academies and a fellow of the American College of Emergency Physicians and the American College of Medical Informatics. He has been chairman of the National Committee on Vital and Health Statistics, and served on the Council on Maternal, Infant and Fetal Nutrition, the Advisory Committee to the Director of the U.S. Centers for Disease Control and Prevention, and the IOM Committee on Assuring the Health of the Public in the 21st Century. He has served on the boards of directors for the Public Health Foundation and the NQF, as president of the Illinois College of Emergency Physicians and the Society of Teachers of Emergency Medicine, and as speaker and board of directors member of the American College of Emergency Physicians. He has received the Arthur McCormack Excellence and Dedication in Public Health Award from the Association of State and Territorial Health Officials, the Jonas Salk Health Leadership Award, and the Leadership in Public Health Award from the Illinois Public Health Association. Dr. Lumpkin also has been the recipient of the Bill B. Smiley Award, the Alan Donaldson Award, the African American History Maker, and Public Health Worker of the Year of the Illinois Public Health Association. He is the author of numerous journal articles and book chapters.

Vimla L. Patel, Ph.D., D.Sc., FRSC, is a senior research scientist at the New York Academy of Medicine and an adjunct professor of biomedical informatics (BMI) at Columbia University in New York. Previously she was a professor of BMI and co-director at the Center for Cognitive Informatics and Decision Making in the School of Biomedical Informatics at the University of Texas Health Science Center in Houston. From 2007-2009, she served as interim chair and vice chair of the BMI department in the Ira A. Fulton School of Engineering at Arizona State University, moving from Columbia University in New York. She has also served on the faculty at McGill University as a professor in the Department of Medicine, and as the director of the Centre for Medical Education, as well as the director of the Cognitive Science Center. She was an elected fellow of the Royal Society of Canada (Academy of Social Sciences), the American College of Medical Informatics, and the New York Academy of Medicine. She was a recipient of the annual Swedish "Woman of Science" award in 1999. She received an Honorary Doctor of Science degree from the University of Victoria in 1998, in recognition of her contributions through cognitive studies in the domain of health informatics. She is an associate editor of the *Journal of Biomedical Informatics* and sits on the editorial boards of *Artificial Intelligence in Medicine* and *Advances in Health Science Education.* She is a past assistant editor of *AI in Medicine* and has served on the editorial boards of *Medical Decision Making,* the *Journal of Experimental Psychology,* and *Computers in Biology and Medicine.* She has served as vice-chair of AMIA's 2009 Scientific Program Committee, vice-chair (membership) of the International Medical Informatics Association, and chair of the editorial committee for *MedInfo* 2001. As a leader in adapting methods/theories from cognitive science and in innovating new approaches that provide scientific foundation for medical education, her research includes the role of cognition in designing a safer clinical workplace. Her studies focus on complexity of the distributed cognitive system that underlies critical care decisions, generation of medical errors, and on the impact of technology on human cognition for competent performance. After moving to the United States in 2000, she became the principal investigator on two R01 awards (from the National Library of Medicine and the National Institute of Mental Health) and on additional awards from the National Library of Medicine and the National Cancer Institute. Currently, she directs a major 5-year James S. McDonnell Foundation research project on Complexity and Error in Health Care with a focus on patient safety. She is a prolific writer with more than 250 scholarly publications spanning biomedical informatics, education, clinical, and cognitive science journals.

Philip Schneider, M.S., FASHP, is clinical professor and associate dean for academic and professional affairs for the University of Arizona, College of Pharmacy at the Phoenix Biomedical Campus. His prior 33 years at Ohio State University included directing the Latiolais Leadership Program at the Ohio State University, an interprofessional program to advance leadership in pharmacy and improve the medication use system to reduce adverse drug events. Mr. Schneider was selected as the recipient of the 2008 Harvey A. K. Whitney Award, known as health-system pharmacy's highest honor, for his outstanding contributions to the practice of pharmacy in health systems. In 2006, he was presented with the Donald E. Francke Medal for significant international contributions to health-system pharmacy. He is a past president of the American Society of Health-System Pharmacists, and past president of the American Society for Parenteral and Enteral Nutrition, having served for 10 years as the first editor-in-chief of *Nutrition in Clinical Practice*, one of its official publications. Active in international pharmacy, he is currently vice president and co-chairman of the Centennial Programme Committee of the Board of Pharmaceutical Practice of the International Pharmaceutical Federation (FIP). Mr. Schneider received a B.S. in pharmacy from the University of Wisconsin, an M.S. in clinical hospital pharmacy from the Ohio State University, and a certificate of residency from the Ohio State University Hospitals. During his 40 years of professional and academic service, he has published more than 170 articles and abstracts in professional and scientific journals, 38 book chapters, edited 7 books, and given more than 500 contributed or invited presentations in 22 countries and the United States.

Christine A. Sinsky, M.D., FACP, is a general internist at Medical Associates Clinic and Health Plans in Dubuque, Iowa. She is a director on the American Board of Internal Medicine, serves on the physician advisory panel for the NCQA physician recognition programs, is a member of the Society of

General Internal Medicine's patient centered medical home (PCMH) working group, and is a consultant for the John D. Stoeckle Center for Primary Care Innovation at the Massachusetts General Hospital. Dr. Sinsky is a frequent invited lecturer on practice innovation, redesign, and the PCMH including for the American College of Physicians, IHI, the Patient Centered Primary Care Collaborative, as well as private and academic medical centers. Dr. Sinsky received her B.S. and M.D. degrees from the University of Wisconsin, Madison, and completed her postgraduate residency and was chief resident at Gundersen Medical Foundation/La Crosse Lutheran Hospital in LaCrosse, Wisconsin.

Paul C. Tang, M.D., M.S., is an internist and vice president, chief innovation and technology officer at the Palo Alto Medical Foundation, and is consulting associate professor of medicine (biomedical informatics) at Stanford University. Dr. Tang is vice chair of the federal Health Information Technology Policy Committee and chair of its Meaningful Use Work Group. Established under the 2009 American Recovery and Reinvestment Act, the group advises the U.S. Department of Health and Human Services on policies related to health information technology. An elected member of the IOM, Dr. Tang chaired an IOM patient safety committee, which published reports in 2003 and 2004: *Patient Safety: A New Standard for Care* and *Key Capabilities of an Electronic Health Record System.* He is also a member of the IOM Board on Health Care Services. Dr. Tang chairs the NQF's Health Information Technology Advisory Committee and is a member of the NQF Consensus Standards Approval Committee. Dr. Tang is a past chair of the board for the American Medical Informatics Association. He is a member of the National Committee on Vital and Health Statistics (NCVHS) and co-chair of the NCVHS quality subcommittee. Dr. Tang co-chairs the measurement implementation strategy work group of the Quality Alliance Steering Committee and chairs the Robert Wood Johnson Foundation's National Advisory Council for ProjectHealth Design. He has published numerous papers in medical informatics, especially related to EHRs, PHRs, and quality, and he has delivered more than 280 invited presentations to national and international organizations and associations. Dr. Tang is a fellow of the American College of Medical Informatics, the American College of Physicians, the College of Healthcare Information Management Executives, and the Healthcare Information and Management Systems Society.

STAFF BIOGRAPHIES

Samantha M. Chao, M.P.H., is a senior program officer and study director at the IOM, where she has primarily worked on issues related to health care quality and patient safety. She has directed studies resulting in the reports *Redesigning Continuing Education in the Health Professions* and *HIV and Disability: Updating the Social Security Listings*. Previously, she directed the Forum on the Science of Health Care Quality Improvement and Implementation, which brought together leaders in the field to discuss methods to improve the quality and value of health care through the strengthening of research. She previously staffed the Pathways to Quality Health Care Series, which reviewed performance measures to analyze health care delivery, evaluated Medicare's Quality Improvement Organization Program, and assessed pay for performance and its potential role in Medicare. Prior to joining the IOM, she completed an M.P.H. in health policy with a concentration in management at the University of Michigan School of Public Health. As part of her studies, she interned with the American Heart Association.

Pamela Cipriano, Ph.D., is the 2010-2011 Distinguished Nurse Scholar-in-Residence at the IOM. As an accomplished hospital and nursing executive, she has led multiple patient care departments at academic medical centers for the past 20 years. She served as chief nursing officer and chief clinical officer of the University of Virginia Health System from 2000 to 2009 and currently holds a faculty appointment as research associate professor at the University of Virginia School of Nursing. She is also editor-in-chief of *American Nurse Today*, the official journal of the American Nurses Association. Dr. Cipriano chaired the American Academy of Nursing's Workforce Commission, studying technology solutions to improve the work environment to make patient care safer and more efficient. Throughout her career, she has been a leader in national nursing organizations addressing issues of policy, administration, quality, technology, and clinical practice. She currently serves on The Joint Commission's National Nursing Advisory Council and the National eHealth Collaborative Board.

Roger C. Herdman, M.D., was born in Boston, Massachusetts. He graduated from Phillips Exeter Academy in 1951; earned a B.S. from Yale University, magna cum laude, Phi Beta Kappa, in 1955; and earned his M.D. from Yale University School of Medicine in 1958. He interned at the University of Minnesota, and was a medical officer with the U.S. Navy from 1959 to 1961. Thereafter, he completed a residency in pediatrics and continued with a medical fellowship in immunology/nephrology at Minnesota. He held positions of assistant professor and professor of pediatrics at the University of Minnesota and the Albany Medical College between 1966 and 1979. In 1969, he was appointed director of the New York State Kidney Disease Institute in Albany. During 1969-1977, he served as deputy commissioner of the New York State Department of Health and was responsible for research, departmental health care facilities, and the Medicaid program at various times. In 1977, he was named director of New York State's Department of Public Health. From 1979 until joining the U.S. Congress's Office of Technology Assessment (OTA), Dr. Herdman was a vice president of the Memorial Sloan-Kettering Cancer Center in New York City. In 1983, he was named assistant director of OTA and then acting director and director from January 1993 to February 1996. After the closure of OTA, he joined the IOM as a senior scholar, and subsequently served as director of the National Cancer Policy Board and the National Cancer Policy Forum. He is now the director of the Board on Health Care Services.

Jensen N. Jose, J.D., is a research associate for the Board on Health Care Services at the IOM. Prior to joining the IOM, Mr. Jose held the position of legal intern at FDA, Office of the Ombudsman, where he assisted in handling complaints and issues against FDA. Mr. Jose received his B.S. in biology and B.A. in political science from the University of Washington in 2007 and received his J.D. from the University of Maryland in 2010.

Herbert S. Lin, Ph.D., is chief scientist at the computer science and telecommunications board, NRC of the National Academies, where he has been study director of major projects on public policy and information technology. These studies include a 1996 study on national cryptography policy (*Cryptography's Role in Securing the Information Society*), a 1991 study on the future of computer science (*Computing the Future*), a 1999 study of Defense Department systems for command, control, communications, computing, and intelligence (*Realizing the Potential of C4I: Fundamental Challenges*), a 2000 study on workforce issues in high technology (*Building a Workforce for the Information Economy*), a 2002 study on protecting kids from Internet pornography and sexual exploitation (*Youth, Pornography, and the Internet*), a 2004 study on aspects of the FBI's information technology modernization program (*A Review of the FBI's Trilogy IT Modernization Program*), a 2005 study on electronic voting (*Asking the Right Questions About Electronic Voting*), a 2005 study on computational biology (*Catalyzing Inquiry at the Interface of Computing and Biology*), a 2007 study on privacy and information technology (*Engaging Privacy and Information Technology in a Digital Age*), a 2007 study on cybersecurity research (*Toward a Safer and More Secure Cyberspace*), a 2009 study on health care informatics (*Computational Technology for Effective Health Care: Immediate Steps and Strategic Directions*), a 2009 study on offensive information warfare (*Technology, Policy, Law, and Ethics Regarding U.S. Acquisition and Use of Cyberattack Capabilities*), and a 2010 study on cyber deterrence (*Proceedings of a Workshop on Deterring Cyberattacks: Informing Strategies and Developing Options for U.S. Policy*). Prior to his NRC service, he was a professional staff member and staff scientist for the House Armed Services Committee (1986-1990), where his portfolio included defense policy and arms control issues. He received his doctorate in physics from MIT.

Joi D. Washington is a research assistant for the IOM Board on Health Care Services. Prior to joining the IOM in May 2008, Ms. Washington held the position of registrar at the National Minority AIDS Council in which she oversaw the registration process for two large national conferences. Ms. Washington received her B.S. in public and community health from the University of Maryland, College Park, in 2007 and is currently pursuing a dual master's degree in health care administration and business administration from the University of Maryland, University College.